舌　　诊

（汉英对照）

Tongue Diagnosis

（Chinese-English）

辛　瑛　郭霞珍　张莉莎　主编

天津科技翻译出版公司

图书在版编目(CIP)数据

舌诊(汉英对照)/辛瑛,郭霞珍主编;张莉莎译 .—天津:天津科技翻译出版公司,2001.5 (2002.4重印)
ISBN 7-5433-1167-4

Ⅰ.舌... Ⅱ.①辛...②郭...③张... Ⅲ.舌诊-图谱-对照读物-汉、英 Ⅳ.R241.25-64

中国版本图书馆 CIP 数据核字(2001)第 05437 号

出　　版: 天津科技翻译出版公司
出 版 人: 邢淑琴
地　　址: 天津市南开区白堤路 244 号
邮政编码: 300192
电　　话: 022-87893561
传　　真: 022-87892476
E - mail: tsttbc@public.tpt.tj.cn
印　　刷: 天津市宝坻县第二印刷厂印刷
发　　行: 全国新华书店
版本记录: 787×1092 32 开本 7 印张 188 千字
2001 年 6 月第 1 版 2002 年 4 月第 2 次印刷
印数:3001－6000 册
定价:28.00 元

作者名单

中文主编　辛　瑛　郭霞珍

编　　者　（按姓氏笔画排名）

丁福康　王玉明　吉凤霞

辛　瑛　宋天彬　郭霞珍

董连荣　梁　嵘

英文主编　张莉莎

翻　　译　张莉莎　倪　健　陈志泰

杨凤勤

英文主审　陈志泰

医学摄影　陈雅洁

Name List of Authours

Chief Authors of Chinese

Xin Ying Guo Xiazhen

Authors (In the Order of Name)

Ding Fukang Wang Yuming

Ji Fengxia Xin Ying

Song Tianbin Guo Xiazhen

Dong Lianrong Liang Rong

Chief Anthour of English

Zhang Lisha

Translators

Zhang Lisha Ni Jian

Chen Zhitai Yang Fengqin

Chief Reviser

Chen Zhitai

Medicine Photographer

Chen Yajie

前　言

舌诊是中医学诊断疾病的一个客观方式。它通过医生对患者舌体变化的观察，对内脏的生理和病理状态做出分析和推断，为临床诊治提供依据。现代研究也认为，舌面仅仅覆盖一层半透明黏膜，就好像一个外露的内脏，是观察人体内在脏腑功能变化的窗口，能客观地反映体内许多生理和病理变化，显示出当时人体的反应性和机能状态，携带着丰富的生命活动信息。舌诊是中医一种已经沿用了两千多年的既客观又便捷的疾病诊断方法。它包括舌神、舌色、舌形、舌态，以及苔色和苔质6个方面。为了满足初学中医者和社区家庭保健的需要，我们从最形象直观的舌象彩图入手，结合临床疾病的诊疗，采用中英文对译的方式，把舌诊知识介绍给中外学者和各位朋友，供大家参阅。

Preface

The inspection of the tongue is an objective way for disease diagnosis. It made analysis and inferences to internal organs through a doctor's observation to a patient's tongue body. The modern research considers that the tongue surface is covered by only a layer of semitransparent mucosa. It seems to be an internal organ which can be seen. It is a window through which you can observe changes of organs' function in a patient's body. It can objectively reflect many physiological and pathologic changes in the body and show then reactivity and function condition in the body. It has a lot of information on life and activity.

The inspection of the tongue is an objective and convenient way for disease diagnosis, which has been used for over 2,000 years in the traditional Chinese medicine. It includes 6 parts, such as the tongue's spirit, color, shape, status and coating's color, fur proper. In order to meet the need of traditional Chinese medicine students and family health in communities, we use the Chinese-English way and introduce the knowledge on the inspection of the tongue to Chinese and foreign students and friends, beginning from the most vivid and objective colored tongue picture, combining the clinical diagnosis and treatment for diseases.

目　录(Contents)

第2部分 临床篇
PART TWO CLINIC

绪 论

中国医药学是一个伟大的宝库。历代医家在长期的临床实践中,创立了许多行之有效的诊察疾病的方法,如"望诊"、"闻诊"、"问诊"、"切诊",舌诊即是望诊中的重要内容之一。

舌诊,又称"望舌",是通过观察舌象(舌质、舌苔等)以了解人体生理功能和病理变化的一种诊察方法。

一、舌诊的起源

中医舌诊的历史可以追溯到距今三千多年前的殷商时代,大约始于西周时代,至春秋战国、秦汉时期已基本形成。我国现存的第一部医学经典著作《黄帝内经》涉及舌诊的内容主要有舌的解剖、生理功能、舌的病理及临床的诊断意义等舌诊知识。主要有诊察舌质、舌苔和舌觉三个方面的内容。

二、汉唐时代舌诊的发展

汉唐时代中医舌诊理论进一步与临床实践相结合,并在实践中不断得到验证、充实和发展。东汉著名医家张仲景(150 年~219 年),把舌诊作为他临床辨证论治法则的一个重要组成部分，并广泛运用于临床诊治中。他认为：其病在表，正气未衰，故多实证热证，诊舌的重点在舌苔变化；内因为患，其病在里，多为虚证寒证，诊察的重点在舌质。

两晋至隋唐时期，舌诊的发展较为缓慢。其中值得一提的有：西晋的王叔和(256 年～316 年)在其所著的《脉经》保存了三国以前的许多舌诊文献，具有很高的史料价值。葛洪、巢元方也比较重视辨舌诊病。巢元方在《诸病源候论》中记载了许多对舌体变化的观察，如舌肿、舌强、舌烂、舌不收、舌缩、弄舌、舌胀、舌出血等；关于舌色苔色的描述也不少，如舌上白、舌上黄、舌焦黑、舌赤、舌青……在诊察病源时，他常把舌象作为疾病的证候之一，给后人以启示。

唐代舌诊也有一些成就，如孙思邈(581 年～682 年)在《备急千金要方》中提出舌象变化属“病在脏腑”的理论，为后世察舌辨脏腑提供了理论根据。

三、宋金元时代舌诊的成就

宋金元时期，是祖国医学全面发展、创立新理论的时代。宋代前期由于社会比较稳定，因而经济有较大发展，科学技术获得了突出的进步，变法后，宋代改革派的革新思潮，也直接影响着医学界，出现了许多著名的革新家，他们总结了以往的经验，提出了新的见解和认识，活跃了学术空气，故而在理论上有许多突破，临证上也取得了许多重要成果。北宋末到元代，社会动荡，战乱不已，疾病流行。社会的需要，成为推动医学发展的直接动力，舌诊在这一时期有了长足的发展，达到了前所未有的水平。

四、明清时期的发展概况

明末至清代中叶，是祖国医学温病学正式确立并逐渐趋于成熟的时期。温病学确立的标志包括了病因学、发病学、病机理论、诊断方法及治疗原则等均有别于伤寒，“温病察舌、伤寒辨脉”就是它们在诊法上的区别。温病察舌起于吴又可，发展完善于叶天士、薛生白、吴鞠通、王孟英等医家，尤其是叶天士、吴鞠通二人创立的一套适用于温热病的辨舌方法，把舌诊与“卫气营血辨证”、“三焦辨证”结合成为一个整体，从而奠定了温病察舌辨证论治的原则。叶天士将舌象变化与卫气营血辨证紧密结合在一起，使舌诊成为温热病辨证论治的主要客观依据，他通过“扪”、“擦”、“问”等具体方法，辨卫、气、营、血，察津液存亡，区别证候。叶氏诊舌法，极受后人重视，吴鞠通在此基础上，结合自己的经验另加发挥，他把舌诊运用于归纳温病属性、辨别三焦病位、指导用药、观测预后等方面，成为三焦辨证(辨湿热病法)的一项重要指标，有一定创造性。

简而言之，舌诊与温病学之间的关系是：温病学的发展推动了舌诊的研究，舌诊所取得的巨大成果又反过来加速了温病学的发展。

应当指出的是，明清迄民国期间，除了温病学对中医舌诊所做的突出贡献外，这一时期还有大量的舌诊著作层出涌现，仅专著专书就达十多种，充分反映出舌诊学发展到这一阶段已基本趋于成熟，临证经验也已相当丰富。其中图谱类专著有申斗垣的《伤寒观舌心法》、张登的《伤寒舌鉴》、王文选的《舌鉴》、梁玉瑜的《舌鉴辨证》、曹炳章的《彩图辨舌指南》，有文无图的舌诊专书有徐灵胎的《舌鉴总论》、傅耐寒的《舌胎统志》、刘恒瑞的《察舌辨证新法》、杨云峰的《临证验舌法》等。此外，还有一些通俗入门普及式的舌诊专著，如陈景岐的《辨舌入门》、缪宏仁的《舌诊学》、何舒的《舌诊问答》等。至于一些综合性医书中所列的舌诊专篇，则更为浩繁，总数逾百。舌诊学在明清至民国时期的大发展，从中可见一斑。

五、中华人民共和国成立后舌诊的整理与研究

建国五十年来，随着中医事业的发展和中西医结合工作的开展，舌诊研究取得了许多可喜的成绩，主要表现在中医教育、研究机构的建立、理论刊物的创办、舌诊文献的大规模整理和新著作的出版，以及对舌诊进行的大量的临床观察等方面。其中最为突出的成就是中西医工作者运用现代科学如血液流变学、血液动力学、微循环、

病理学、细胞学、生物化学、免疫学、微量元素分析、舌色仪等多种实验手段对中医舌诊——这一古老的诊法进行深入研究，从而使舌诊在客观化、规范化方面取得了很大进展。这些科学研究验证并补充了以往的舌诊理论，基本阐明了舌质与舌苔形成的原理及其变化的部分因素，初步掌握了临床常见疾病的舌象变化规律，并将此作为某些疾病（如感染性疾病、心血管疾病、肿瘤等）的重要诊断指标，从而使舌诊成为中医独特并与现代科学相结合的诊断方法之一。

由于舌诊具有重要的诊断价值，且无创伤，方便易行，故舌诊这种古老的诊法在诊断和辩治疾病方面将会有更广阔的前景，而且，随着科学技术的发展，它将会不断地焕发出新的更加强大的生命力。

Introduction

The traditional Chinese medicine is a great treasure house. In the long clinical practice, doctors in successive dynasties created many efficient disease diagnostic ways, for example, inspection, auscultation and olfaction, interrogation, and pulse taking and palpation. The tongue diagnosis is an important content in the method of inspection.

The tongue diagnosis is also called the inspection of the tongue. It is a diagnostic way to understand the physiologic function and disease changes in the human body by observing the tongue phenomenon (tongue proper and tongue coating, etc.).

Ⅰ. The origin of the inspection of the tongue

The inspection of the tongue in the traditional Chinese medicine can be traced back to the Yin-Shang era over 3,000 years ago. Almost it was basically formed in Xizhou, Chunqiu, Zhanguo, Qin and Han dynasties. The earliest traditional Chinese book *huang di nei jing*《黄帝内经》began to concern the knowledge on the dissection, physi ological function and clinical importance of the tongue. In it, there is a content in 3 areas including the tongue proper, tongue coating and tongue sense.

Ⅱ. The development of the inspection of the tongue in Han and Tang dynasties

In Han and Tang dynasties, the theory on the inspection of the tongue in the traditional Chinese medicine was further combined to the clinical practice. It was demonstrated, replenished and developed in the practice.

Zhang Zhongjing(A. D. 150 – 219), a famous doctor in Donghan Dynasty, considered the inspection of the tongue as an important part in his differentiation of symptoms and signs as well as clinical treatment, and widely used it in his clinical treatment. He said, the disease could be reflected on the surface, vital Qi was not weak, as a result, you could see real signs and heat syndromes. The key in the inspection of the tongue was at the coating of the tongue. The internal factor would be the main factor. The disease was in the human body. The key for the inspection was at the tongue proper.

During the two Jins to Sui and Tang dynasties, the development of the inspection of the tongue was slow. One which was worthy to be mentioned is the man of the west Jin Dynasty Wang Shuhe (A. D. 256 – 316). The book *Canon of Pulsology*《脉经》, which was written by him, reserved many documents that were before the three Nations. Those documents have high value in the history. The other two were Ge Hong and Cao Yuanfang. They paid more attention to the inspection of the tongue as well. Cao Yuanfang recorded some observations of changes of the tongue body in his work *General Treatise on the Cause and Symptoms of Diseases*《诸病源候论》, such as swelling of the tongue, stiffing of the tongue, rotting of the tongue, loosening of the tongue, shortening of the tongue, continuously moving tongue, expanding of the tongue and bleeding of the tongue. Moreover, there were many descriptions of the colors of tongue body and tongue coating, such as white coating of the tongue, yellow coating of the tongue, black and dye coating of the tongue, reddened tongue, bluish tongue. When he looked for the cause of a disease, he always regarded the picture of the tongue as one of syndromes of the disease, which enlightened his following men.

There were also a few achievements in the inspection of the tongue during Tang Dynasty. For an example, Sun Simiao (518 – 682 A.D.) put forward in his work *Prescriptions Worth a Thousand Gold for Emergencies*《备急千金要方》that the changes of the picture of the tongue should belong to the theory of diseases in zang-organs and fu-organs, which offered a theoretical basis for descendent on inspecting tongue to different viscera.

Ⅲ. Acheivements of inspection of the tongue during Song Dynasty, Jing Dynasty and Yuan Dynasty.

The period of Song, Jin and Yuan dynasties is the era when the traditional Chinese medicine developed comprehensively. Because of the stability of the Song Dynasty's society, the economy developed very fast. Moreover, the science and technology made prominent progress. After changing laws, the innovative trend of thought of Song renovations made a direct effect on medicine. Many famous renovations emerged. They summarized previous experience and put forward new opinions and views, which enlivened the scientific atmosphere and caused many breakthroughs in the theory. The innovation also led to many important achievements in the clinic. During the time from late North Song to Yuan Dynasty, the society was turbulent and wars broke out constantly, which caused diseases spread. Needs of society became the direct power promoting the medical development. And the inspection of the tongue also made rapid progress during the time and reached an unprecedented level.

Ⅳ. Acheivements of inspection of the tongue during Ming Dynasty and Qing Dynasty.

The subject on seasonal febrile diseases of traditional Chinese medicine was formally established and gradually became a mature subject during the period from the late Ming Dynasty to the middle period of Qing Dynasty. Ye Tianshi, founder of this subject, made changes of pictures of tongues as the main objective basis of diagnosis and treatment based on overall analysis of symptoms and signs to epidemic febrile diseases. By touching, brushing, inquiring, he analyzed and studied the conditions of the Four Syndromes Wei, Qi, Ying and Xue and body fluid, so as to distinguish the syndromes. Ye's method of the inspection of the tongue is highly valued by the following people, however, Wu Jutong made another use of this method by combining his own clinic experience. He put the inspection of the tongue to use in the following ways: summing up the categories of febrile diseases, differentiating syndromes according to pathological changes of the triple – Jiao, guiding to use medicine, and foreseeing diseases' result. It is creative for him to make the inspection of the tongue an index of the differentiation of syndromes according to the pathological changes of the triple-Jiao, which is the method of analysis of symptoms and signs to dampness-heat diseases.

We must mention that a lot of works on the inspection of the tongue came out from Ming and Qing Dynasty to Mingguo, which also contributes a lot to the development of the inspection of the tongue besides the outstanding contribution that the subject of seasonal febrile diseases has made. Special books even amounted to over ten categories, it fully reflected that the development of the inspection of the tongue had come near to a mature stage and that the clinic experience had been rather abundent. Among the books, the following are with pictures: *shang han guan she xin fa*《伤寒观舌心法》by Shen Douyuan, *shang han she jian*《伤寒舌鉴》by Zhang Deng, *she jian*《舌鉴》by Wang Wenxuan, *cai tu bian she zhi nan*《彩图辨舌指南》by Cao Binzhang; the following are with no pictures: *she jian zong lun*《舌鉴总论》by Xu Lingtai, *she tai tong zhi*《舌胎统志》by Fu Naihan, *cha she bian zheng xin fa*《察舌辨证新

法》by Liu Hengrui, *lin zheng yan she fa*《临证验舌法》by Yang Yunfeng, etc. There were also some ABC books on the inspection of the tongue, such as *bian she ru men*《辨舌入门》by Chen Jingqi, *she zhen xue*《舌诊学》by Liao Hongren, *she zhen wen da*《舌诊问答》by He Shu. Moreover, over hundreds of articles on the inspection of the tongue can be found in many synthetical medical works. In a word, we can see the development of the subject of the inspection of the tongue from all above.

Ⅴ. Arrangement and research of the inspection of the tongue after the P.R.C was founded

Along with the development of the traditional Chinese medicine (TCM) and integrated work of TCM with the western medicine, great achievements have been made in the research of the inspection of the tongue in the past 50 years after the People's Republic of China was founded. The outstanding one is the researchers in TCM and western medicine, which carried on further research on the inspection of the tongue of TCM, an old diagnostic method, using modern scientific experimental technique, such as hemodynamics, microcirculation, pathology, cytology, biochemistry, immunology, microelement analysis. It makes great progress on objectifying and standardizing the inspection of the tongue. These researches verified and complemented previous theories on the inspection of the tongue, and basically clarified the developing principles and some changing factors of the inspection of the tongue. They also obtained the changing laws of the picture of the tongue that was seen in usual clinical diseases and regarded the laws as some diseases' important diagnostic standards. It made the inspection of the tongue as one of the diagnostic methods that combined traditional Chinese medicine with modern science.

Because the inspection of the tongue not only has important diagnostic value and has no pain but also is convenient, it will own more development prospect on diagnostics and treating diseases. Moreover, with the development of scientific techniques, the inspection of the tongue will show constantly fresh and stronger living power.

第 1 部分　基础篇
PART ONE　BASIS

望舌主要包括望舌质、望舌苔二部分内容。舌质，又称舌体，即舌的肌肉脉络组织；舌苔是附着于舌面上的一层苔状物。

中医传统诊法认为，舌质与舌苔在反映病证方面各有侧重，一般来说，舌质多反映五脏精气的盛衰，舌苔多反映病邪的性质及病位的深浅。这是因为舌质的色泽形态主要是依靠五脏所化生的精气上荣以维持，故五脏精气的盛衰也就主要表现在舌质上；舌苔由胃气上蒸而成，若体内有邪气，常与胃气相互搏结上蒸于舌面，而表现为舌苔的异常，故舌苔更侧重于反映病邪的情况。由于中医发病学理论更注重正气的盛衰，故相比较而言，中医望舌更注重舌质的变化。

望舌质又可细分为望舌神、望舌色、望舌形、望舌态四个方面。

望舌苔，是望舌面上的那层苔状物。舌苔是舌象的重要组成部分，有重要的临床意义，尤其是对了解胃气的有无、胃津的存亡、病邪的性质，以及推断病情的轻重等，意义更为重大。望舌苔，包括望舌苔的"形质"和望舌苔的"颜色"两个方面。中医学认为，人之所以有舌苔，是"胃中生气"的表现，是由"胃蒸脾湿上潮而生"，所以，正常的健康人都有一层薄薄的白色舌苔。如果人体发生病变，邪气就会与胃气相抟结，上蒸于舌面就会出现异常的舌苔。

The inspection of the tongue comprises two parts: the tongue body and tongue coating.

The traditional Chinese medicine considers that the tongue body and coating can reflect pathogenic conditions respectively in different ways. Generally speaking, the tongue body mainly reflects the sufficiency or deficiency of vital Qi in the viscera, while the coating reflects the nature of pathogen as well as the depth of disease location. For the tongue property is nourished and supported by vital Qi that is from the viscera, and the coating is formed by upward steaming action of the stomach Qi, which is often complicated by pathogens inside the body. Between the two parts, the inspection of tongue is comparatively important in observation of the tongue, since vital Qi has more significance in disease occurrence according to the traditional Chinese medical theory.

In detail, inspection of the tongue includes four parts: (1) inspection of the tongue spirit; (2) inspection of the tongue color; (3) inspection of the tongue shape; (4) inspection of the tongue state.

Inspection of the coating means to observe the layer of fur like substance on the tongue surface. The tongue coating is an inseparable part of a tongue picture, and it is of great importance in clinic, especially in detecting conditions of the stomach Qi and fluid, or nature of pathogens, as well as in judging severity of pathological condition.

Observation of the coating contains two aspects: the fur proper and its color. In TCM opinion, the fur is a manifestation of the stomach vital Qi, for it is formed by upward steaming of the stomach Qi upon the spleen fluid. Therefore the healthy body can present a layer of thin and white coating. If any illness occurs, pathogenic factors will ascend together with the stomach Qi up to the surface of the tongue, and develop an abnormal fur.

第1章 望舌神

舌神主要表现在舌质的荣润和灵动方面。“荣润”是有活生生的光彩，“灵动”是运动灵活。望舌神可以统领舌色，凡有神舌无论舌色如何，都为“活色”，凡无神舌无论舌色如何，均为“死色”。如红舌，有神的红舌其色泽红活荣润，无神的红色则色泽晦暗如猪肝。

Chapter 1 Inspection of the Tongue Spirit

The tongue spirit can be showed in two aspects: (1) vitality, (2) mobility. The vitality means lively color and luster of the tongue, while the mobility means freedom of movement. In the inspection, the tongue spirit is considered to be in charge of the tongue color. The tongue with spirit refers to "lively color", no matter what kind of color it is. The tongue without spirit refers to "death color". For example, a red tongue with spirit will appear fresh color and moisture. But without spirit it will be lusterless, dim and dark, similar to the liver of a pig.

一、有神舌（图1.1）

【舌象】舌质荣润而有光彩，舌色红活，运动灵敏，充满生气。

【机理】舌之有神，说明五脏功能正常，化生精气充盛，胃气未伤，气血能够上荣于舌，故表现出神采外露。

Ⅰ. The Tongue with Spirit (Figure 1.1)

【Manifestations】The tongue proper is glossy, moist and lively colored, free to move, and full of vitality.

【Mechanism】The tongue with spirit is formed as a result of normal function of the viscera, which can transform sufficient essence Qi and send Qi and blood up to the tongue for good nourishment.

二、无神舌

【舌象】舌质干枯而晦暗无泽，死板而毫无生气，运动失灵。

【机理】舌质无神，说明五脏功能衰竭，精气匮乏，或胃气衰败，气血不能上荣于舌，故表现为神气全无，临证见此舌象，说明正气大伤，“诸病皆凶”。

Ⅱ. The Tongue without spirit

【Manifestations】The tongue is dry, dim and lusterless. Its body loses flexibility and freedom of movement.

【Mechanism】The tongue has no spirit, indicating exhaustion of the viscera activities, essence Qi, as well as the stomach Qi. Under such a condition, Qi and blood can not be sent upward to the tongue for nourishment, manifested as no vitality on the tongue at all. When this kind of tongue pictures is seen in clinic, it reflects heavy impairment of vital Qi and unfavorable prognosis of diseases.

第2章 望舌色

舌色是指舌质的颜色，临床将舌色分为淡红、淡白、红、绛、紫、青六种，其中除淡红舌为正常舌色外，其余均为主病之舌色。

Chapter 2 Inspection of the Tongue Color

The tongue color refers to colors of tongues, including light red, pale, red, crimson, purple, and blue in clinic. Among them, all colors are abnormal except light red color.

一、淡红舌（图1.1）

【舌象】舌色不深不浅，红活润泽。

【机理】淡红舌是脏腑气血上荣之色，标志着脏腑机能正常，血液充盛，阳气和畅，阳气鼓动血液在体内运行，反映于舌部，即可见舌色淡红荣润。所以，淡红舌为正常健康人的舌色，也见于一些患轻微小病及病情较轻的患者。

【主病】表证温邪初起，实证、热证和虚证之较轻者。

Ⅰ. The Light Red Tongue (Figure 1.1)

【Manifestations】The color of tongues is neither dark nor light, showing light red, lustrous and moist.

【Mechanism】A light red tongue is the color of tongue nourished by Qi and blood of the viscera, and a sign of normal function of the Zang-Fu organs. It is a result of exuberant blood and harmonious Yang Qi that drives blood flowing around the body, reflected by the light red, lustrous and moist tongue. So the light red tongue is the healthy color, or occurring in some mild illness.

【Indications】It indicates onset of the exterior syndrome by warm pathogen, as well as mild cases of excessive syndrome, heat syndrome, or deficient syndrome.

二、淡白舌(图 2.1)

淡白舌之舌色比正常舌要浅淡，白多红少，甚则枯白全无血色。淡白舌的形成机理为虚、寒。虚，是指气血不足，不能充斥血络；寒，是指阳气不足，不能温运血液上荣于舌，又阳虚则内寒，血脉收引，使舌部血量减少，故见舌色淡白。淡白舌是中医辨证"虚寒证"或"气血两虚证"之典型舌象，常见于现代医学疾病中的各种贫血，严重的营养不良或一些慢性疾病。

临床常见淡白舌及主病如下。

Ⅱ. The Pale Tongue(Figure 2.1)

The tongue is pale and lighter than normal, looking more white and less red, or even deadly pale without blood color at all. The reason is deficiency or cold. Deficiency refers to both Qi and blood insufficient, failing to fill up blood vessels. Cold refers to insufficiency of Yang Qi, which can not warm and drive blood upward to the tongue for nourishment, bringing the tongue pale in color. Moreover, deficient Yang can lead to interior cold that makes blood vessels' contraction, reducing blood volume of vessels, manifested as pale tongues. The pale tongue is the typical tongue picture of deficient cold syndrome, or deficient syndrome of both Qi and blood, often seen in cases of anemia, severe malnutrition, and some chronic diseases.

Pictures of tongues commonly seen in clinic as well as their indications are as follows.

1. 淡白瘦薄舌(图 2.2)

【舌象】舌色淡白，舌体小于正常而见瘦薄，苔多为薄白或较少，舌面无过多水分。

【主病】气血两虚。气血虚少，不能充斥血管脉道，所以舌色浅淡而舌体瘦薄尖削。由于气血衰少，机体各部失养，所以患者常有疲乏无力，声低息微，心悸自汗，气短懒言，面色、爪、口唇色淡，头晕目眩，耳鸣时作，脉虚细无力或微细无力等症。

【治法】双补气血。

1. The Thin and Pale Tongue(Figure 2.2)

【Manifestations】 The tongue is pale and thinner than normal. The coating is mostly thin or less, without much fluid on the surface.

【Indications】 Deficiency of both Qi and blood. Qi and blood are insufficient, failing to fill up blood vessels of the tongue, leaving the tongue pale in color and thinner in shape. Because of deficiency of Qi and blood, the every parts of body are malnutrition, giving rise to lassitude, low voice, palpitation, spontaneous sweating, short of breath, pale complexion, pale lips and nails, dizziness, blurred vision, tinnitus, weak and thready pulse, etc. This kind of conditions can be seen in terms of western medicine as anemia, extreme malnutrition, chronic renal disease, some severe or prolonged illness, or weak constitution.

【Treatment】 To strengthen Qi and replenish blood.

2. 淡白胖嫩齿痕舌(图2.3)

【舌象】舌色淡白,舌体胖嫩,舌边多有齿痕,苔多白腻或水滑。

【主病】脾肾阳虚、水湿内停。这种舌象形成的机理主要是因机体阳气不足,特别是脾肾阳虚,以致水液代谢失常,水湿内停所致。体内水湿过多,水气上溢,舌体因而胖大而湿润水滑。同时,脾肾阳虚也会使血液的生成和运行不利,所以舌色变淡。脾肾阳虚水湿内停常见畏寒肢冷,小便不利,浮肿,嗜睡,腹胀便溏,口泛清水,脉象沉迟无力等症状。

【治法】温补脾肾,兼以利湿。

2. The Pale, Enlarged and Tender Tongue with Tooth Prints(Figure 2.3)

【Manifestations】 The tongue is pale, puffy, and tender with tooth prints on its border. The coating is white, sticky and sticky, or even watery.

【Indications】 Retention of water dampness due to yang deficiency of the spleen and kidney. The deficient spleen and kidney yang can not promote water metabolism normally, resulting in stagnation of water dampness which flow upward to the tongue, leaving the tongue body enlarged and shown moisture or watery. Meantime the condition of yang deficiency can also affect normal production and circulation of blood, bringing the tongue pale in color. The syndrome of yang deficiency in the spleen and kidney is often manifested by aversion to cold, cold limbs, disuria, edema, sleepiness, abdominal distention, loose stool, profuse clear saliva in the mouth, deep, slow and weak pulse, etc.

【Treatment】 To warm and reinforce the spleen and kidney combined with excreting dampness.

3. 淡白舌,白腻干苔(图 2.4)

【舌象】舌质淡白,舌面少津,苔白干裂,中有两条厚腻苔。

【主病】阳气虚损,气化失司;湿阻中焦,津不上承。多由于阳气虚损不能化生津液,或不能很好地布散津液而成,也可由于湿阻中焦,影响津液的输布,津不上承所致。

【治法】扶阳益气,化气行水。

3. The Pale Tongue with Dry, White and Sticky Fur(Figure 2.4)

【Manifestations】 The tongue is pale and less moist, covered by the white, dry and fissured coating with two pieces of thick stick coatings in the middle.

【Indications】 Yang is deficient and dysfunctional in generation or distribution of body fluid, resulting in obstruction of the middle-Jiao by stagnant fluid which fails to flow upward onto the surface of the tongue.

【Treatment】 To warm yang and benefit Qi, in order to distribute body fluid.

4. 淡白夹红舌(图 2.5)

【舌象】舌淡胖嫩,舌边尖部较红,或舌尖部有红点,苔多为白润或淡黄薄腻。

【主病】脾虚湿滞化热。脾气虚运化失司,水湿停留体内,日久化热,故苔多淡黄而腻。

【治法】健脾益气,清热利湿。

4. The Pale Tongue with Red Parts(Figure 2.5)

【Manifestations】 A tender, enlarged and pale tongue is red in its edges and tip or has red spots in the tip. The coating is white, moist, or thin, yellowish and sticky.

【Indications】 This kind of tongue pictures results from the spleen deficiency and dampness heat of the interior. Since the spleen is insufficient, it fails to transform and transport water dampness, which accumulates in the interior and consequently turns into heat. As a manifestation, the coating is yellowish and sticky.

【Treatment】 To invigorate the spleen Qi and clear away dampness heat.

5. 淡白光莹舌(枯白舌)(图 2.6)

【舌象】舌色淡白,毫无生气,舌苔全部脱光,好像新剥皮的鸡肉一样,故又被称为"光莹舌"、"枯白舌"。

【主病】阳气虚极,气血枯竭,主危重病证。枯白舌属无神淡白舌,说明脏腑阳气已近衰竭,气血已不能上荣于舌,"必连龈、唇皆无血色"。

【治法】温补阳气,补气生血。

5. The Pale and Glossy Tongue(Withered White Tongue)(Figure 2.6)

【Manifestations】 The tongue is pale without any vitality. The coating is peeled off entirely, just as a chicken whose skin is newly peeled, which is described as "a glossy white tongue" or "withered white tongue".

【Indications】 Decline of Yang, exhaustion of Qi and blood, indicating the critical stage of diseases. The withered white tongue belongs to the pale tongue without vitality, indicating exhaustion of Yang Qi in the viscera. Qi-blood can not be sent upward to the tongue for nourishment, bringing about a withered tongue picture.

【Treatment】 To warm and strengthen yang Qi, or to reinforce Qi and replenish blood.

6. 淡白偏暗舌(图 2.7)

【舌象】舌质色淡而暗滞,舌形较胖,边有齿痕,苔白腻,根部有腐苔。

【主病】气虚湿阻血瘀。如果阳气不足,不能推动和温煦血行,就会导致血行滞涩不畅。此外,阳虚气化不利多生寒湿,寒湿邪气阻遏气血的运行并可进一步损伤阳气,也可致血行不畅,故见舌色淡暗,实为气虚湿阻而血行不畅。

【治法】补益阳气,温化寒湿。

6. The Pale and Dim Tongue(Figure 2.7)

【Manifestations】The color of the tongue body is pale and dark. The shape of the tongue is puffy with some tooth prints on the sides. The coating is white and sticky, showing some curdy coating in the root part.

【Indications】 Yang deficiency, retention of dampness, and blood stasis. Since Yang is deficient, it can warm and promote neither blood circulation nor water metabolism, leading to stagnation of blood as well as retention of cold dampness. Cold dampness may obstruct the flow of Qi-blood, and it can further injure Yang Qi in turn resulting in stagnation of blood as well. This can be learnt through the pale and dim tongue. The tongue is a sign of Qi deficiency and dampness obstruction as well as blood stagnancy.

【Treatment】To warm and strengthen Yang Qi for resolving cold dampness.

三、红舌(图 2.8)

舌色比正常舌红,称为红舌。因血得热则行,热盛则气血沸涌,舌体血脉充盈,故舌色变红。舌色越红,提示热邪越重。

临床常见红舌及主病如下。

Ⅲ. The Red Tongue(Figure 2.8)

The tongue with red color darker than normal is termed a red tongue. Since blood circulates when it gets heat, heat excess can drive blood flowing rapidly and violently, leaving blood vessels fullness and bringing the tongue red in color. The redder the tongue shows, the more serious the heat evil is.

The red tongue commonly seen in clinic as well as their indications are as follows.

1. 舌边尖红(薄白苔)(图2.9)

【舌象】舌质大部分为正常色，舌边尖部偏红，苔白左边较厚。

【主病】温热袭表，邪犯肺卫。因邪气在表，里热未盛，故舌色变化还不大或略偏红，或仅限于局部。常伴有表证常见之症状，如微恶风寒，发热，头痛，咽喉痛，咳嗽、四肢酸痛，脉浮数等。

【治法】辛凉解表。

1. The Tongue With Red Sides and Tip (Thin White Fur) (Figure 2.9)

【Manifestations】 The tongue is mostly normal in color, but its sides and tip show light red. The coating is white and thick coating can be seen in the left part.

【Indications】 Invasion of the exterior by warm heat, and attack of the lung-Wei system by exogenous pathogen. Since the pathogen still remains at the exterior, the interior heat is not excessive. Therefore the tongue color has less change, or only appears light red, or red limited partially. It is often accompanied by symptoms commonly seen with the exterior syndrome, such as slightly aversion to wind-cold, fever, headache, sore throat, cough, sourness and aches in the four limbs, and floating rapid pulse, etc.

【Treatment】 To relieve the exterior syndrome with acrid-cool herbs.

2. 舌红(苔黄厚干燥)(图2.10)

【舌象】全舌红赤，红色鲜明，苔黄厚干裂少津。

【主病】里热炽盛。此舌象在外感病、内伤病中均可见到。在外感病，多为温热邪气入里进入气分，或其他外邪入里化热(如寒邪从阳化热等)；在内伤病，主要见于各脏腑的火热证，如心火、肝火、肺火、胃火等。无论外感或内伤，此时的病机特点均为邪气亢盛，正气也不衰，正邪交争剧烈，导致脏腑机能亢奋而呈现一派阳热有余的实热征象。热迫血妄行，气血沸涌，自里达表，故外现全舌红赤；又由于热邪熏蒸，所以舌苔多黄厚；热盛伤津，故舌苔干燥。主要临床表现可见壮热汗出，面红目赤，心烦口渴，渴喜冷饮，大便干燥，小便短赤，脉数有力等。

【治法】清热生津。

2. The Red Tongue (with the Yellow, Thick and Dry Fur) (Figure 2.10)

【Manifestations】 The whole tongue shows red and fresh. The coating is yellow, thick and dry with fissures.

【Indications】 It denotes excessive heat in the interior. This kind of tongues may be seen in both exogenous diseases and internal injury diseases. In exogenous diseases, it is caused by pathogenic warm-heat that has transmitted into the internal Qi-system from the exterior, or by the interior heat transformed from other exogenous pathogens (such as cold pathogen, changing into heat under influence of yang constitution). In interior injury diseases, it occurs within some internal fire heat syndromes of the viscera, such as heart fire, liver fire, lung fire, and stomach fire. At this stage, no matter the exterior or interior syndrome it is, pathogen is intense with vital Qi no deficiency. They struggle against each other fiercely, leading to hyperactivity of the viscera function, showing excessive heat syndrome of Yang exuberance. Heat pathogen forces blood to circulate rapidly so as to make blood vessels fully filled, therefore producing a fresh red tongue. Furthermore the excessive heat steams upwards and damages the body fluid, causing a thick, yellow and dryness coating. The main symptoms linked with this tongue are as follows: high fever, sweating, red face and eyes, restlessness, thirst with preference to cold drinks, constipation, scanty dark urine, rapid and forceful pulse, etc.

【Treatment】 To clear away heat and produce body fluid.

3. 舌红偏暗(苔焦黄、灰黑)(图2.11)

【舌象】舌红偏暗，舌质苍老，舌苔焦黄灰黑，干糙裂纹。

【主病】胃肠热结(阳明腑实),气血壅滞;三焦实热伤阴。这种舌象常由上一舌象进一步发展而成。由于热邪过盛伤津,而致燥屎内结,阻滞气机,邪热被闭郁于内不得外达,致使气血壅滞,故舌红偏暗,内热不得外泄伤津越甚,故舌苔由黄厚变为焦黄、焦灰、焦黑。主要临床症状可见高热不退,大便秘结不通,腹满胀痛,面红息粗,潮热汗出,烦躁不宁,甚则神昏谵语,脉沉实有力。

【治法】急下存阴;泻下清热。

3. The Red, Slight Dark Tongue (Covered by Dark Yellow, or Gray Black Fur)(Figure 2.11)

【Manifestations】The tongue is dark red and rough. The coating is dark yellow, grayish black and dry with fissures.

【Indications】It suggests heat obstruction in the gastrointestinal tract, and stagnation of Qi-blood; or exhaustion of yin fluid by excessive heat of three-Jiao.

This kind of tongues is developed from the former one. Since the heat pathogen is over abundant and impairs body fluid. It can cause retention of dry stools in the interior, which may obstruct the activity of Qi, leaving pathogenic heat blocked in the interior. Heat pathogen fails to reach the exterior, as a result, both Qi and blood is stagnated. So the dark red tongue is formed. The internal heat can not exit outsides, and damages the body fluid more severely, bringing the coating color turned from yellow, thick to dark yellow, dark gray, or even dark black color. The main disorders can be high fever, constipation, distending pain in the abdomen, flushed face, rough breath, tidal fever with sweating, restlessness, even a coma and delirium, deep and forceful pulse.

【Treatment】To purge bowels urgently for saving yin fluid, or to purge and eliminate heat pathogen.

4. **舌红(苔黄腻)(图 2.12)**

【舌象】舌质红,苔黄而粘腻。

【主病】湿热痰涎内结。此种舌象是热邪与痰涎湿浊交结而成,其形成原因或由于热邪太甚炼液成痰,或素有痰湿又邪热炽盛,凡属痰热证、湿热证多见此舌象,如痰火所致的狂证、中风、眩晕、不寐、咳、哮、喘等，以及肝、胆、脾胃、大肠、膀胱等脏腑的湿热证。

【治法】清热化痰；清热利湿。

4. The Red Tongue (with Yellow and Sticky Fur) (Figure 2.12)

【Manifestations】The tongue is red. The fur is yellow and sticky.

【Indications】It is attributable to the interior stagnancy of dampness heat and phlegm. This type of tongue pictures results from heat pathogen complicated with phlegm fluid and dampness turbidity. The formation is due to either heat pathogen hyperactivity so as to scorch the body fluid into phlegm, or phlegm dampness existing previously again suffering from excessive pathogenic heat. In clinic, the tongue picture is usually seen in syndromes of phlegm heat, and dampness heat, such as mania due to phlegm fire, wind-stroke, dizziness, insomnia, cough, asthma, and some disorders in the liver, gallbladder, spleen-stomach, large intestine, and urinary bladder, etc.

【Treatment】To clear away heat and resolve phlegm, or to eliminate heat and excrete dampness.

5. 舌红(少苔)(图 2.13)

【舌象】舌质红，舌体瘦，舌苔少。

【主病】阴虚内热。此为虚热舌象，在外感病中多为热邪初退，津液大伤，一时还未能恢复；在内伤病，多见于各脏腑的阴虚火旺证，如心阴虚、肝阴虚、肺阴虚、肾阴虚、胃阴虚等。阴液亏少不能充斥舌体，故舌体多变得瘦小或瘦薄；津亏不能上潮于舌面长养舌苔，故舌苔少，严重者甚至不能成苔而见舌光剥无苔。

【治法】养阴清热。

5. The Red Tongue (with Less Fur) (Figure 2.13)

【Manifestations】The tongue is red in color and thin in shape. The coating is less.

【Indications】It suggests the interior heat due to Yin deficiency. This is a tongue picture of deficient heat. In the case of exogenous syndrome, it indicates newly retreated heat pathogen with heavy injured body fluid that hasn't restored. In the case of internal injury, it results from hyperactive fire of Zang-Fu organs due to Yin deficiency, such as the heart Yin deficiency, the liver Yin deficiency, the lung Yin deficiency, the kidney Yin deficiency, and the stomach Yin deficiency, etc. Yin fluid is not sufficient enough to supply the tongue for nourishment, bringing the tongue body smaller and thinner than normal. For the same reason, the coating is less, or even no coating at all.

【Treatment】To replenish Yin and reduce fire.

四、绛舌

绛,为深红色,主病有外感与内伤之分,并有虚实之辨。在外感病,绛舌的出现标志着热邪进入营分,内伤病绛舌多见于阴虚火旺,临床常见绛舌,其主病如下。

Ⅳ. The Crimson Tongue

The tongue is dark red. The indications include exogenous and endogenous diseases. In the exogenous one, it means invasion of the Ying-system by pathogenic heat, while in the endogenous one, it suggests hyperactivity of fire due to yin deficiency. The crimson tongues commonly seen in clinic and their indications are as follows.

1. **绛舌少苔**(图 2.14)

【舌象】舌质红绛鲜泽,有裂纹,无苔少津。

【主病】热伤营阴;阴虚火旺。此舌象为外感温热病热入营分的典型舌象。温热邪气初入营分,其势甚张,营血内炽,血热蒸腾,故舌色比红舌更深,又因热伤营阴,津液亏乏,所以常见苔少或无苔。此期常见发热以夜晚为重,口渴反不如气分证重,心烦躁扰,或有少许斑疹出现等症状。

绛舌少苔也可见于内伤杂病,多为阴虚火旺的严重疾病。

【治法】清营透热;滋阴降火。

1. The Crimson Tongue with Less Fur(Figure 2.14)

【Manifestations】The tongue is crimson and fresh, showing fissures, less moisture, and no coating.

【Indications】It is a typical tongue picture of heat invading Ying-system in the exogenous febrile disease. The pathogenic heat has just invaded the Ying-system and it is extremely intense. Heat pathogen disturbs Ying-blood, leading to violent circulation of blood, which brings the tongue into dark red color. Simultaneously, pathogenic heat injures Ying-Yin, and consumes the body fluid, giving rise to a tongue without coating or with less coating. In this period some symptoms are commonly seen such as fever pronounced in the evening, less thirst than that in Qi-system, restlessness, delirium, or some eruptions, etc.

This kind of tongues can also occur in miscellaneous diseases of internal injury. It indicates severe diseases due to hyperactive fire and yin deficiency.

【Treatment】To clear Ying-system and expel heat, or to nourish yin and reduce fire.

2. 红绛光莹舌(图 2.15)

【舌象】舌质红绛,舌上无苔,光亮如镜面,望之似有光泽,扪之干燥无津,质地不苍老反见娇嫩。

【主病】胃阴大伤或胃阴亡失。这种舌象在外感病主要见于温热病后期热灼胃津,导致胃阴大伤甚则胃阴亡失;内伤病则多见于一些慢性消耗性疾病的晚期,此舌属危重舌象,说明胃气胃阴大伤,已不能上蒸于舌面而形成舌苔,其病多重笃。

【治法】滋补胃阴。

2. The Crimson and Glossy Tongue(Figure 2.15)

【Manifestations】The tongue is crimson. There is no coating on the tongue. It is as glossy as a mirror, and feels dry without fluid. The property of the tongue is not rough but tender.

【Indications】Severe damage or exhaustion of the stomach yin. It can be seen at the late stage of seasonal febrile diseases if it occurs in exogenous cases. Heat pathogen is burning the stomach fluid, leading to heavy injury or exhaustion of the stomach yin. It can also be seen at the late stage of some chronic consumptive cases if it occurs in interior injury diseases. It is a critical sign, meaning that the serious consumed stomach Qi and yin can not steam upward onto the tongue to form the tongue coating. Diseases linked with that are usually critical.

【Treatment】To nourish the stomach yin.

3. 红绛晦暗枯瘦舌(图 2.16)

【舌象】舌质红绛而色泽晦暗,舌体瘦小,干瘪枯痉,舌面干燥少津无苔,舌体可见颤动。

【主病】肝肾阴竭。这种红绛晦暗枯瘦的舌象多由阴虚火旺之红绛少苔舌发展而来,中医学认为肾阴为一身阴液之根本,故无论外感病还是内伤病,凡见此舌象,标志着肝肾之阴已涸竭,证属危候,舌象也为危重舌象。

【治法】滋阴熄风。

3. The Dark Crimson and Emaciated Tongue(Figure 2.16)

【Manifestations】The tongue is crimson and dark. The tongue body is thin, shortened, and withered. It is dry and has no coating on the surface of the tongue. The body of the tongue can be seen trembling.

【Indications】Exhaustion of yin in the liver and kidney. This kind of tongues is developed from the crimson with less coating tongue that is due to hyperactive fire and yin deficiency. In TCM opinion, the kidney yin is the root of yin-fluid in the whole body. So it typifies exhaustion of yin within the liver and kidney, belonging to a critical case, no matter occurring in the exogenous disease or in internal injury diseases.

【Treatment】To nourish yin and stop wind.

五、青紫舌

青舌、紫舌虽均示血行不畅,血液瘀滞,但主病却与前面所述的淡白舌、红绛舌不同,淡白舌主虚主寒,红绛舌主热,均主性质相同的一类病证,而青紫舌则不然,青紫舌可主性质截然相反的两种病证——寒证和热证。寒证青紫舌以青为主兼有紫色。这类舌的舌苔多湿润,甚则水气不化而见舌苔水滑。热证的舌色则为绛紫、深紫,这种舌色是从红绛舌发展而来的,这类舌的舌面多干燥少津。临床常见青紫舌及主病如下。

Ⅴ. The Blue-Purple Tongue

The blue-purple tongue results directly from stagnation of blood that can be caused by both cold and heat. So the tongue can indicate either cold syndrome or heat syndrome. This is different from the pale or red crimson tongue, for the pale tongue indicates the syndromes of deficiency and cold, while the red crimson tongue suggests the disease of heat. They indicate the same kind of syndrome respectively. But the blue-purple tongue can suggest two opposite syndromes, cold and heat. When manifesting cold syndrome, the blue-purple tongue is mainly blue, marked with moisture or even watery. When manifesting heat syndrome, the tongue is crimson purple or dark purple. It is developed from the red crimson tongue, and the surface is usually less moist and dry. The blue-purple tongues and their indications commonly seen in clinic are as follows:

1. **紫绛舌(图 2.17)**

【舌象】全舌紫绛,实热证多有黄、灰、黑干燥苔;虚热证则苔少或无苔。本照片,为营热夹湿,舌上仍有薄苔。

【主病】血分热毒深重。可见,紫绛舌主热极,是从红绛舌发展而成的,标志着病入血分,是外感温热病发展的最严重阶段。临床常有神昏、谵语、动血(吐血、呕血、便血、尿血、皮下出血紫黑)、动风(惊厥抽搐)等症状。

【治法】凉血散血(散血:滋阴活血)。

1. The Purple-Crimson Tongue(Figure 2.17)

【Manifestations】The whole tongue shows purple crimson. It can be covered either by the yellow, gray, black and dry coating when occurring in excessive heat syndrome, or by less coating and even no coating if in deficient heat syndrome. The picture as above has the thin coating because of heat in the Ying-system complicated with dampness.

【Indications】The toxic heat of the blood-system is very serious. The purple crimson tongue means extremely heat, developed from the red crimson tongue. It indicates invasion of blood system by pathogenic heat, manifesting the most critical period in the seasonal febrile disease. The symptoms, such as coma, delirium, bleeding (hematemesis, nasal bleeding, bloody stools, hematuria, skin purpura.), convulsions, are commonly seen in clinic.

【Treatment】To cool the blood and dissipate blood stasis.

2. **紫晦舌(图 2.18)**

【舌象】舌质紫绛,但不鲜泽,晦暗无光,毫无生气,如同猪肝色,光剥无苔,舌体痉软不能伸缩,或颤抖不已,语言不利。

【主病】肝肾阴竭,亡阴失水。此舌象在外感温热病或内伤杂病中都为肝肾阴竭之象,其病证多危重。临床常见形体高度消瘦,皮肤干皱,唇焦舌萎,目陷睛迷,两颧红赤,心悸作痛,手足微微抽搐或抖动,甚则神昏嗜睡,脉微细欲绝等阴精大伤的症状。

【治法】滋阴养血,潜阳熄风。

2. The Crimson and Dim Tongue(Figure 2.18)

【Manifestations】The tongue is purple crimson, dim, no luster and vitality. It is similar to the liver of a pig, with the coating all peeled off. The tongue body is too flaccid to extend, or too tremulous to speech clearly.

【Indications】The tongue as above can be seen in the exogenous warm-heat disease or internal injury disease, being a sign of yin exhaustion of the liver and kidney, and indicating a severe condition. Clinically the symptoms such as emaciation, dry skin and lips, red cheeks, palpitation, trembling limbs, even unconsciousness, and feeble pulse, etc., due to heavy injury of yin essence, may present.

【Treatment】To nourish yin and replenish blood, combined with suppressing yang and reliving convulsion.

3. **淡白青紫舌(图 2.19)**

【舌象】舌质在淡白的基础上略见青紫,舌上滑润。也有见舌淡有瘀斑、瘀点者。

【主病】寒凝血瘀。此舌象是由淡白舌发展而成,寒为阴邪,具有凝滞收引的特性,血遇寒则凝,血脉收引拘挛，血液运行不畅，故呈现此种舌象。

【治法】散寒化瘀。

3. The Pale and Bluish Purple Tongue(Figure 2.19)

【Manifestations】 The tongue is slightly bluish purple on the base of pale color, and it is moist. In some cases, the pale tongue can be complicated with petechia.

【Indications】 The tongue indicates blood stasis due to cold. It is developed from the pale tongue. Since cold belongs to yin pathogen, it has the property of coagulation and contraction. Blood circulation can be coagulated when exposured to cold, and contraction and spasm of the blood vessels may arise. Unsmoothed flow of blood gives rise to the tongue like this one.

【Treatment】 To dissipate cold pathogen and remove blood stasis.

4. 紫暗瘀斑瘀点舌(图 2.20)

【舌象】舌质紫暗色滞，多处见瘀斑。也有的舌象见舌边尖部有瘀斑瘀点。

【机理】血液流行不畅，甚至瘀塞不通而形成瘀血。当瘀血形成后，又可成为一种新的病因作用于人体，产生更为复杂更为严重的病变，形成各种瘀证(如瘀血阻心、瘀阻胞宫、瘀阻经络、瘀阻清窍……)。青紫舌还可见于药物、食物中毒及酒毒等。

4. The Dark Purple Tongue With Blue Spots(Figure 2.20)

【Manifestations】 The tongue is dark and purple without luster. Some blue or purple spots can be seen on its border and tip.

【Indications】 This tongue picture typifies blood stasis. When blood circulation is unsmooth or even obstructed, it can further develop to blood stasis, which becomes a new pathogenic factor to act upon the body in turn. And then some more complicated and serious disorders may appear, such as cardiovascular diseases, uterus disorders, obstruction of meridians, cerebral vascular diseases, and so on. Moreover, the bluish purple tongue can also occur in cases of alcoholism, poisoning of food or medication, etc.

第3章 望舌形

舌形、舌态的变化，也是内在脏腑气血发生寒、热、虚、实病理变化的反映，所以，望舌形、望舌态也应像望舌神、舌色一样，注意观察了解全身整体的情况，要四诊合参，更应注意结合舌色、舌苔的变化，将这些情况综合起来加以分析研究，这对于正确地辨证施治是至关重要的。

舌形的异常变化常见的有以下几种。

Chapter 3　Inspection of the Tongue Shape

Changes of the shape and state of tongue reflect the pathology of Qi and blood in cool, heat, and weak or excess stage. So the correct differentiation is based on overall analysis of the patient's symptoms, signs, physical conditions, and especially the shape and state of tongues. This chapter is about the shape and state of tongues, which is similar to the color and expression of tongues in another chapter.

Common abnormal changes of the shape of tongues are as follows.

一、苍老舌(图3.1)

【舌象】舌质纹理粗糙，形色坚敛。舌质苍老是舌色与舌形的综合表现，如舌色深暗，舌上起刺或裂纹，或舌质纹理粗糙干燥皱缩等。

【机理】《辨舌指南》说："凡舌质坚敛而苍老，不论苔色黄、白、灰、黑，病多实证。"由于邪正交争剧烈，气血壅盛，反映于舌即见舌色红赤有根底，甚则出现芒刺，纹理不细腻(即所谓"老"象)。故苍老舌主实证、热证。

【主病】邪气亢盛。

【治法】祛除邪气。

Ⅰ. The Bleak and Dark Tongue(Figure 3.1)

【Manifestations】 The bleak and dark tongue means the tongue texture with slipshod lines. This is the combined appearance of the shape and color of tongue. Forexample, the tongue is dry, dark, covered with rough lines and has some thorns or cracks on it.

【Mechanism】 *Bian she zhi nan* (a Guide to Differentiation of Tongues) says: "Hard and bleak tongues belong to excess symptom no matter what color they are, like yellow, white, gray or black". The reason for this is the struggle between vital Qi and pathogenic factor.

【Indications】 Excess of evil Qi.

【Treatment】 To dispel the evil Qi.

二、娇嫩舌(图 3.2,3.3)

【舌象】舌质纹理细腻,浮胖娇嫩。舌色或淡白无华(图 3.2),或色红娇艳(图 3.3)。

【机理】《辨舌指南》指出:"舌质浮胖兼娇嫩,不拘苔色黄、白、灰、黑,病多属虚。""虚",是指正气虚,"虚证",是指人体的机能活动(包括脏腑、经络、气血等功能)和抗病、康复能力低下,临床表现为一系列虚弱、衰退和不足的证候。虚热证由于阴不制阳,虚热内生,所以,舌质在娇嫩的基础上可见色红而娇艳。

【主病】正气不足(阳气不足,阴液亏损)。

【治法】补益正气(补益阳气,滋阴降火)。

Ⅱ. The Tender Tongue(Figure 3.2,3.3)

【Manifestations】 The tender tongue means the tongue texture is puffy with fine and smooth lines. Its color is pale or fresh red.

【Mechanism】 *Bian she zhi nan* says: "Puffy and tender tongues belong to deficiency syndrome no matter what the color they are, like yellow, white, gray or black". Deficiency syndrome refers to the morbid condition showing deficiency of genuine Qi, lowered body resistance, declining of function etc. All these are the clinical deficiency signs. For the fever of deficiency type that is caused by weak of yin, yin can not control yang, giving rise to deficient heat, so the tender tongue shows bright red.

【Indications】Deficiency of vital Qi, including yang deficiency and-yin fluid deficiency.

【Treatment】To invigorate vital Qi, including the treatment of invigorating yang and nourishing yin to reduce pathogenic fire.

三、胖大舌(图3.4)

【舌象】舌色淡白、舌体胖嫩,比正常舌体大而厚,甚则充满口腔。舌上多津水滑。

【机理】这种舌象的形成主要是由脾肾阳虚,气化失常,水湿内停,上泛于舌而成。如舌象与上述相同,但舌尖部嫩红,或见有淡黄腻苔,说明有虚阳上浮或湿郁化热存在,治疗时应兼顾引火归原和利湿清热。

【主病】脾肾阳虚,水湿内停。

【治法】补益阳气,化气利湿。

Ⅲ. The Big and Fat Tongue(Figure 3.4)

【Manifestations】The tongue texture with over saliva is bigger and thicker than the normal one, even filling the mouth. The color of the tongue is pale.

【Mechanism】This condition of the tongue is mainly caused by insufficiency of both the spleen and kidney-yang, which leads to abnormal transformation of Qi, resulting in retention of water dampness. It floats upward, and brings in the tongue watery. If the tongue as above but red at the tip or showing light yellow coating, it means upward floating of deficient yang or attack of fire caused by damp stagnancy. So the treatment way should pay attention to these two aspects and adapt as conducting fire back to its origin and eliminating dampness heat accordingly.

【Indications】Insufficiency of both the spleen and kidney yang.

【Treatment】To reinforce yang-Qi for transformation of Qi and excreting dampness.

四、肿胀舌

【舌象】舌体肿胀,严重者可因过度肿胀而不能缩回口中。舌肿胀与舌胖大不同,多由邪热太盛或中毒所致,分述如下。

Ⅳ. The Swollen Tongue

【Manifestations】 The tongue is swollen and can not be withdrawn into the mouth in the serious case. This is different from the big and fat tongue. It is mainly caused by excessive heat or poisoning. Details are as follows.

1. 鲜红肿胀舌(图 3.5)

【舌象】舌肿胀灼热疼痛,舌色红绛鲜泽。边尖有红点。

【机理】这种舌象多见于心脾(胃)有热,使气血上壅,如伴有神志不清,更足以证明热入心包,心火上炎,气滞血壅;若舌红肿胀满布黄腻苔垢,多为湿热蕴毒上泛。

【主病】心脾热盛或感湿热毒气。

【治法】清泻心脾积热;清热利湿解毒。

1. The Fresh Red Swollen Tongue(Figure 3.5)

【Manifestations】 The swollen tongue shows red or dark red color, some red clots at the tip. Patients have feeling of burning pain.

【Mechanism】 This condition is usually caused by upward stagnancy of Qi and blood due to pathogenic heat in the heart, spleen and stomach. If heat pathogen attacks the pericardium, the heart-fire will flame upward and cause stagnation of Qi and blood, giving rise to unconsciousness. Accumulation of dampness-heat in the body often results in red, swollen tongue covered with yellow coatings.

【Indications】 Excessive heat in the heart and spleen, or attack by dampness-heat and toxic Qi.

【Treatment】 To clear away pathogenic heat of the heart and spleen; or to clear away heat and excrete dampness, as well as to remove toxin.

2. 青紫肿胀舌(图 3.6)

【舌象】舌紫而肿或色紫黯而发青,口唇也肿大而青紫。

【机理】这种舌多见于中毒,如酒毒和食物、药物中毒等,毒物造成血液凝滞而见此舌象。严重的瘀血,也可见到此舌象。

【主病】中毒、瘀血。

【治法】解毒、化瘀。

应注意有先天性舌血管瘤患者,也可见舌的局部肿胀色紫,但无辨证意义,临证时应注意除外这种情况。

2. The Swollen Tongue in Black Purple Color(Figure 3.6)

【Manifestations】The swollen tongue and lips show purple or dark purple color.

【Mechanism】This condition is found in the case of intoxication, like alcoholism, food or drug poisoning, which leads to abnormal circulation of blood, bringing the tongue in darkness. It may also be caused by serious blood stasis.

【Indications】Intoxication or blood stasis.

【Treatment】Detoxification; Removing blood stasis. This condition of tongue may also occur in cases of congenital tongue hemangioma.

五、瘦薄舌

舌体比正常舌瘦小而薄,称为"瘦薄舌"。舌体是由肌肉、血脉等组织组成,气血不足,舌肌瘦削,舌体必现瘦薄,为舌体不充的表现,故瘦薄舌主气血两虚和阴血不足,分述如下。

Ⅴ. The Thin and Small Tongue

The tongue texture is thinner and smaller than the normal one. This is mainly because of insufficient Qi, blood and yin. Details are as follows.

1. **淡白瘦薄舌(图 3.7)**

【舌象】舌形瘦薄,舌色淡白,甚则枯白无华。

【机理】心主血脉,脾主肌肉,舌的血脉归心所主,舌的肌肉靠脾化生的气血荣养。如心脾两虚,气血生成不足,能充盈濡养舌体,舌体必渐渐瘦薄无华。此种舌象主要见严重的贫血、长期的胃肠功能紊乱、营养不良症，以及一些慢性消耗性疾病等。

【主病】气血大亏。

【治法】补益气血。

1. The Thin and Small Tongue in Light White Color(Figure 3.7)

【Manifestations】The tongue is thin and pale, even withered with white color.

【Mechanism】The tongue is related to the heart and gets nourishment from the spleen, since the heart controls blood vessels and spleen controls muscle. Insufficiency of the heart and spleen will induce the insufficiency of Qi and blood, which leads to the thin and withered tongue. This symptom occurs easily in serious anemia, chronic gastrointestinal dysfunction, nutritional deficiency and chronic consumptive diseases.

【Indications】Severe deficiency of Qi and blood.

【Treatment】To benefit Qi and blood.

2. 红绛瘦薄舌(图 3.8)

【舌象】舌色红绛而舌形瘦薄，少苔。

【机理】这种舌象在外感病热伤营阴和内伤病阴液虚证中均可见到。形成的原因主要是：阴液不足，舌体失充，阴液不足不能制约阳气，故出现阴越伤、火越旺、阴更伤的恶性循环，舌体更现瘦薄，甚则枯瘦干瘪。此种舌象多于外感热病的后期，热伤营阴；内伤病也多见于一些慢性消耗性疾病中医辨证为阴虚火旺的病证，如结核病、癌症、消化系统疾病、糖尿病、甲状腺功能亢进、慢性心肾疾患等。

【主病】阴虚火旺。

【治法】滋阴降火。

瘦薄舌为正气(气血、营阴)虚损舌象，故无论新病、久病，见此舌象，均示病情较重，若枯萎无津或舌色晦黯，是为无神舌，预后尤为不良。

2. The Thin and Small Tongue in Red and Dark Purple Color(Figure 3.8)

【Manifestations】The thin and small tongue appears in red

and crimson color, less coating.

【Mechanism】The main reason is that yin-fluid is deficient and can not control yang-Qi, resulting in hyperactivity of fire due to yin deficiency. So the tongue becomes thinner and smaller gradually because of less nourishment by yin fluid. This tongue picture can occur at the late stage of epidemic febrile diseases caused by exogenous evils, or in some chronic consumptive diseases, such as cancer, tuberculosis, digestive system, diabetes, hyperthyroidism, chronic disease of heart and kidney.

【Indications】Hyperactive fire due to yin deficiency.

【Treatment】Nourishing yin to lower fire.

This picture of tongue is the sign of severe deficiency of Qi, Blood, ying and yin, so it means the illness is at the serious stage. If the tongue is dry, withered, without saliva, and the color is dark, it belongs to "the tongue without spirit", meaning unfavorable prognosis.

六、裂纹舌

舌面上出现各种形状的裂纹、裂沟，深浅不一，多少不等，统称为裂纹舌。舌见裂纹，多属气血阴液亏损，是舌体失于濡养的表现，然而也有实热有此舌者，主要见于心火和胃火炽盛，有报道说瘀血证也可见到此舌，使用活血化瘀药物后，情况得到了改善。

Ⅵ. The Fissure Tongue

The fissure tongue refers to the surface of the tongue covered with all kinds of crackles or lines in deep or shallow shape. This belongs to the deficiency of Qi and blood, the excess fire of heart and stomach. Some books report that this syndrome occurs in blood stasis.

1. 红绛少苔裂纹舌(图 3.9)

【舌象】舌有裂纹，舌色红绛，少苔或无苔光燥。

【机理】据临床观察，此舌象是裂纹舌中最为常见的一种，即阴虚兼有裂纹。其形成机理主要为阴液亏损，不能濡养滋润舌体，故舌生裂纹。常见于外感热病后期热盛伤阴,或内伤杂病阴虚火旺之证。

【主病】阴虚火旺。

【治法】滋阴降火润燥。

1. The Fissure Tongue in Red and Crimson Color, with Less Fur(Figure 3.9)

【Manifestations】The cracked tongue in red and crimson color, showing dry, little or no coating.

【Mechanism】According to clinical observation, this kind of tongue pictures is the most common one among the cracked tongues, i.e. yin deficiency with fissures. This is due to deficiency of yin-fluid, so the tongue receives no nourishment. The deficiency of yin-fluid is usually caused by epidemic febrile diseases, or internal injury diseases marked by hyperactive fire.

【Indications】Hyperactive fire due to yin deficiency.

【Treatment】Nourishing Yin to lower fire.

2. **淡白裂纹舌(图 3.10)**

【舌象】舌色淡白有裂纹;有的舌象淡白胖嫩裂纹满布,边有齿痕。

【机理】这两种舌象略有差别,前者主要由于气血不足,血虚失于濡润而成;后者则多见于脾胃气虚,脾虚湿浸。

【主病】血虚不润;脾虚湿浸。

【治法】养血润燥;健脾利湿。

需要注意的是:裂纹舌有先天禀赋生而即有者,应与病理性裂纹舌相鉴别,前者舌色红活荣润,裂纹长期不变,而由疾病所致者则随病情轻重发生变化。另外,裂纹舌主要是指舌质的裂纹,有时舌苔也随之出现裂纹,但仅舌苔有裂纹者则不属裂纹舌范围。

2. The Fissure Tongue in Pale Color(Figure 3.10)

【Manifestations】The fissure tongue in pale color: some of them are fat, tender with cracks, and showing tooth prints.

【Mechanism】These two types of pictures are similar but have some difference. The former is caused by deficiency of Qi and blood, so the tongue does not receive enough nourishment. The latter is usually seen in the case of Qi-deficiency of both spleen and stomach that causes dampness retention.

【Indications】Deficiency of blood, or spleen insufficiency with dampness accumulation.

【Treatment】To nourish blood and moisten dryness, or to reinforce the function of spleen for removing dampness.

In two aspects we should take notice: one is that some people have inborn cracked tongues. These lines can not change, and color and shape of tongues are normal. It should be differed from the morbid fissure tongues, which can be changed with seriousness of illness. The second is that the tongue texture has lines meaning the fissure tongue, sometimes accompanied by the cracked coating. If the tongue has slits only on the coating, it does not belong to the fissure tongue.

七、齿痕舌(图3.11)

【舌象】舌体的边缘有牙齿的痕迹,舌色多淡白;舌形多胖大,然也有正常或瘦薄者。

【机理】与胖大淡白舌并见者多为脾虚水湿不运,其形成机理与胖大舌相同。舌体正常或瘦薄而见齿痕者,则多为气虚或气血两虚,使舌体不充盈、舌肌张力不足所致。这种舌常见于水肿、贫血、慢性心肾疾患者。

【主病】脾虚湿盛;气血两虚。

【治法】健脾利湿;补益气血。

Ⅶ. The Tongue with Tooth Prints(Figure 3.11)

【Manifestations】At sides of the tongue texture there are tooth prints. The shape of the tongue is usually enlarged but some can be normal or thin. The color of the tongue is pale.

【Mechanism】An enlarged tongue in pale color is mostly caused by the spleen-deficiency. A normal shape of the tongue or the thin tongue with tooth prints is mostly due to the Qi-deficiency or deficiency of both Qi and blood. This can be seen in patients who suffer from edema, anemia, and chronic heart and kidney diseases.

【Indications】Excessive dampness caused by spleen-deficiency, or deficiency of both Qi and blood.

【Treatment】 Invigorating the spleen to eliminate dampness, or nourishing Qi and blood.

八、点刺舌

点色红的称为“红点舌”(图 3.12);色白的称为“白星舌”。

点刺舌,均主热毒炽盛。多见于外感热病热盛极期和内伤杂病脏腑阳热亢盛。临床常见于高热、急性传染病(特别是发疹发斑性疾病,如麻疹、猩红热等)和急性化脓性感染(如化脓性阑尾炎、化脓性胆囊炎、重症肺炎等),以及烧伤、败血症等。临证凡见此舌象,均提示热毒极盛,病情重笃。

根据点刺所生的部位,可以推测邪热所在的脏腑或何脏腑热邪最甚,如舌尖生点刺,多为心火亢盛;舌中生点刺,多为胃肠热极。

根据点刺的颜色和分布的疏密,可以估计热邪的轻重,如点刺鲜红散在,说明血热尚轻;如舌色紫绛芒刺满布,说明血热极盛,病情危重。

白星舌散布于舌中根部,多与红绛舌并见,提示热极伤阴或营养不良。

舌生点刺兼有舌苔者(如黄燥、灰燥、黑燥苔),多为实热内结(气分热极);舌生点刺少苔或无苔者,多为热盛气阴大伤(热入营血)。

Ⅷ. The Dot and Thorn Tongue

The dot and thorn tongue is caused by dominance of noxious heat. “Dot” can be divided into “red dot” which refers to the dot color being red(Figure 3.12), as well as “white dot” which refers to the dot color being white. ”The thorn tongue” can also be called “prickly tongue”. They are often seen at the late stage of epidemic febrile diseases caused by exogenous pathogens or all kinds of inner problems induced by excess of yang. In terms of western medicine, the diseases are high-fever, acute infectious disease (measles and scarlet fever, etc.), acute pyogenic infection (pyogenic cholangitis, suppurative appendicitis, serious pneumonia), phlebitis, infection of burn, etc. When this type of tongues is seen, it indicates that the toxic heat is vigorous and the disease is at serious stage.

According to the location of dots on the tongue, the doctor can infer pathogenic heat in which Zang Fu-organs or where the evil heat is dominant. For example, dots on the tongue tip means hyperactivity of the heart-fire, while dots in the middle of tongue means excessive fire of the stomach and intestinal.

According to color and distribution of the dots and thorns, the doctor can infer whether the problem is mild or serious. For example, if the color of dots and thorns is bright red and scattered, it means the heat of blood is mild. If the color of dots and thorns is dark purple and tightly packed on the tongue, it means the heat of blood is vigorous and the illness is serious.

If there are white dots in the middle of the tongue with a red and crimson tongue body, it indicates consumption of yin by febrile disease, or nutrition deficiency.

If the tongue has thorns accompanied by yellow, gray or black and dry coating, it means accumulation of excess-heat (excessive heat in Qi system). A thorny tongue with little or no coating means heavy impairment of yin due to intense heat (excessive heat in ying and blood system).

1. **红绛芒刺舌(杨梅舌)(图**3.13)

【舌象】舌色红绛,干燥起刺,状若成熟的杨梅。

【机理】热邪极盛,深入血分,热迫血行,气血沸涌,使舌上红粒充血肿大增生突起。临证见此舌象提示血分热毒极盛,也常是动风动血的先兆。

【主病】热入营血,阴液大伤。

【治法】清热凉血,养阴生津。

1. The Thorny Tongue in Red and Crimson Color (Bayberry or Strawberry Tongue)(Figure 3.13)

【Manifestations】 The thorny tongue shows dry, red and crimson color like bayberry.

【Mechanism】 The tongue indicates that extreme heat attacks blood system and causes rapid blood circulation, giving rise to dots and thorns formed on the tongue. It is a sign of convulsion or bleeding.

【Indications】 Extreme heat evil attacking in blood and serious deficiency of yin.

【Treatment】 Removing pathogenic heat from blood and replenishing yin to produce fluid.

2. 红点舌(如前述)(图 3.12)

2. The Red Dot Tongue See above(Figure 3.12).

九、重舌(图 3.14)

【舌象】舌下血络肿起,如舌下又生了一个小舌,与舌体重叠,故称为"重舌"。初发时,舌下血络颜色鲜红、疼痛、活动不利,日久,血络变为青紫色,肿痛减弱。

【机理】此舌多由心经火热,循经上冲,或外邪引动心火上炎而成。临床多见于舌下腺炎、舌下腺囊肿以及肿瘤等。

【主病】心火上炎。

【治法】清心泻火。

Ⅸ. The Double Tongue(Figure 3.14)

【Manifestations】 On the underside of the tongue there is another small tongue because of swollen blood vessels, so this is called the double tongue. At the beginning it is aching and difficult in its movement, showing bright red color. At the late stage the pain is not serious and the color turns to blue purple.

【Mechanism】 The reasons may be fire in the heart channel flaming upward, or exterior evil inducing hyperactive heart-fire. Clinically this can be found in hypoglossiadenitis, abscess of sublingual gland, tumor, etc.

【Indications】 Flaming up of the heart-fire.

【Treatment】 To clear away heart-fire.

十、舌衄(图 3.15)

舌体出血称为舌衄,主要由血热妄行或气不摄血所致。血热妄行又有虚实之分。实热出血颜色鲜红,血量较多,常伴有舌体红肿硬木,多由心脾热盛或胃热熏蒸所致,如舌衄现于舌下,多为肝热迫血。阴虚舌衄多与红绛光剥、裂纹舌同见，舌上出血不多，舌体肿痛也不甚，原自阴虚火旺，虚热迫血。属气虚不摄血者，大多见舌质淡白胖嫩，舌衄主要为渗血不止，并伴有气虚常见的症状，如面色无华，气短心悸，倦怠乏力，脉细弱无力等，临床常见于白血病、再生障碍性贫血等血液病。

【主病】热迫血行；气不摄血。

【治法】实热清热凉血；虚热滋阴降火；气虚不摄血者补气摄血。

Ⅹ. The Bleeding Tongue (Figure 3.15)

The bleeding tongue refers to blood oozing from the tongue. The main reason is heat in blood or Qi failure in controlling blood. There are deficiency and excess types of heat in the blood condition. For the excess type: the color of bleeding is bright red, and volume is large, usually combined with the symptoms of red, swollen, heat and aching in the tongue texture. This is mostly caused by excessive heat in the heart, spleen or stomach. For example, bleeding under the tongue indicates heat in the liver forcing blood out. For the deficient type: bleeding may be caused by yin deficiency. In this case, other signs may occur like glossy tongues in crimson color and fissures, and bleeding or aching of the tongue being mild. It is caused by yin deficiency with hyperactive fire that forces blood out. If it is due to Qi deficiency, the tongue texture will appear pale, tender and enlarged, as well as prolonged oozing of blood, often accompanied with pale complexion, shortness of breath, palpitation, tired, weak pulse etc. This tongue type can be found in leukemia, aplastic anemia, etc.

【Indications】 Heat forcing blood out, or failure of Qi in controlling blood within the vessels.

【Treatment】 To clear away heat and cool blood for excessive type, nourishing Yin to lower fire for deficiency type, homeostasis by tonifying Qi for Qi deficiency type.

十一、舌痈（图 3.16）

【舌象】舌上肿痛，局部根盘较大，初起质硬、溃后流脓。

【机理】火热之邪入于血分，聚于局部，热毒壅滞而肉腐成痈。舌红少苔痈生舌上者，多为心火上炎；舌红或绛，痈生舌下者，多属脾肾积热。临床均属舌的化脓性感染。

【主病】心火上炎；脾肾积热。

【治法】清心泻火；泻热滋阴。

Ⅺ. Abscess of the Tongue(Figure 3.16)

【Manifestations】 Swollen, hard, pain is at onset, followed by formation of the tongue abscess.

【Mechanism】 It is mostly caused by stagnation of toxic material resulting from the hyperactivity of heat-fire and accumulation of heat-evil. Carbuncle appears on the tongue covered by less coating, mainly caused by flaming of the heart fire. The reddish or crimson tongue with abscess under it, is usually caused by the stagnation of heat at the spleen and kidney. All these belong to the pyogenic infection in clinic.

【Indications】 Flaming of the heart fire, or accumulation of heat at the spleen and kidney.

【Treatment】 To clear away the heart fire, or nourishing yin to expel heat.

十二、舌疔（图 3.17）

【舌象】舌上生豆状或樱桃状红、紫色疱，根脚紧缩而深，质地坚硬而剧痛。

【机理】舌疔的形成与舌痈相同，也多为心脾火毒郁滞而成。

【主病】心脾火毒。

【治法】清心凉脾，泻火解毒。

Ⅻ. The Tongue Pustule(Figure 3.17)

【Manifestations】 Manifested as a purplish, hard and painful bean-sized pustule on the tongue.

【Mechanism】 The reason is same as pyogenic infection of the tongue, due to accumulation of fire-evil in the heart and spleen.

【Indications】The fire-toxin at the heart and spleen.

【Treatment】Clearing away fire and expelling the toxic material to cool the heart and spleen.

十三、舌疮(图 3.18)

【舌象】舌上生溃疡,如粟米大小。其证有虚火实火之分。凡心火挟毒者,疮面多凸于舌面,红赤肿痛较剧。虚火者,如阴虚火旺或气虚阳浮,疮面多高起不甚,有的甚至低凹不起,溃面经久不愈,也不太疼痛。临床多见于溃疡性舌炎,常反复发作,经久不愈。

【主病】心火挟毒;虚火上攻。

【治法】实证清热解毒;虚证阴虚者滋阴降火;气虚者扶正托毒。

XIII. Boils of Tongues(Figure 3.18)

【Manifestations】There is erosion on the tongue. The ulcer area looks like millets. For excess type: the surface of the sore is protruding the tongue in red color, swelling, and extremely pain. For deficiency type: the surface of sore is not protruding the tongue obviously. Some of them may be even hollow, and hard to cure, with mild pain. In clinic this can be seen in ulcerative tongue infection.

【Indications】The heat-evil at heart, or flaming up of deficient fire.

【Treatment】For excess type: to clear away heat-toxin, for deficiency type of yin: nourishing yin to lower fire, for Qi deficiency type: supporting the vital Qi to descend heat-toxin.

十四、舌菌(图 3.19)

【舌象】舌生恶肉,初起如豆大,渐渐头大蒂小,好似"泛莲"、"鸡冠"或如"菜花",色红或紫,发展较快,表皮破溃出血,剧痛难忍,流涎极臭,舌体活动受限,甚则波及舌周围组织。初则木硬皮色不变,久则破溃穿腮。

【机理】舌菌的形成原因主要由于七情郁结,心脾郁火,热毒上攻所致,属舌的恶性肿瘤,多预后不良,《灵枢》说:"舌本烂,热不已者死。"

【主病】心脾郁火，热毒上攻。

【治法】清心解毒，去瘀止痛。

XIV. The Carcinoma of the Tongue(Figure 3.19)

【Manifestations】Tumor grows on tongue about the size of a bean at onset, but gradually it shows shapes of "cockscomb" or "cauliflower" or "lotus". The color is red or purple, and it develops rapidly. The surface appears ulcer and bleeding. The patient feels extreme pain. Salivation smells terribly foul. The tongue texture can not move freely. The illness affects surrounding tissues. Secreting from the tumor will eventually cause erosion of the cheek.

【Mechanism】The main causes is the stagnation of seven emotional factors, accumulation of fire in the heart and spleen, and flaming up of heat-evil. It belongs to malignant tumor in clinic. *Ling Su Jing* (miraculous pivot) says: "if there is erosion on the tongue and the fire can not be controlled, it may lead to death".

【Indications】Accumulation of fire at the heart and spleen, and flaming up of heat-evil.

【Treatment】To clear away the heart heat and toxin, and to stop pain by removing blood stasis.

第4章 望舌态

舌态，是指舌体的活动或静止时的状态。正常舌态为舌体柔软、运动自如，无偏歪、颤动等异常活动。当机体发生病变影响或反映于舌时，可引起舌体运动的改变，主要有软、硬、颤、纵、歪、缩、吐弄等。

Chapter 4　The shape of tongue

The shape of the tongue refers to the condition of the tongue texture when it is still or moving. A normal tongue is soft and can move freely. The state of an abnormal tongue can be stiff, trembling, retracting, extended, etc.

一、痿软舌

舌体软弱，伸缩无力，甚则痿废不用，称为“舌痿”。多由气血虚或阴液亏损，以致舌的筋脉和肌肉失养所致。久病舌淡而痿，多是气血双亏；新病舌干红而痿，是热灼津伤；久病舌绛无苔而痿，是阴亏已极。

临床比较常见的痿软舌是红绛少苔瘦薄痿软舌。多见于外感热病的后期热邪伤津耗液、消灼精血，或内伤病久阴液精血大伤，以致舌体失养，瘦弱不用。

【治法】治法滋阴养血。

Ⅰ. The Flaccid Tongue

The symptom refers to the tongue withering and too weak to move freely, caused by damage of Qi, blood and yin-fluid. If this condition occurs for a long time and the tongue is pale, it indicates the deficiency of both Qi and blood. If the tongue recently becomes flaccid and is dry and red, it indicates the consumption of fluid by heat. A flaccid tongue developed over a long period has no coating and dark purple color, it indicates extreme deficiency of yin.

In clinic the most common case is the thin flaccid tongue in red and dark purple color, and little coating. This is mainly found at the late stage of exogenous febrile diseases or internal injury diseases, while the body fluid and blood have been injured, leading to the tongue's less nourishment and inability to movement.

【Treatment】 Nourishing yin and blood.

二、强硬舌(图 4.1)

舌体板硬强直,运动不灵,称为"舌强"。舌强在外感或内伤病中均可见到,在外感病主要见于热入心包证,其机理是:热入心包,炼液成痰,痰热阻塞舌本脉络,加之高热伤津舌体失养,以致舌体失其柔韧之性而见舌强语謇,舌色红绛苔黄腻或干,故《辨舌指南》说:"凡舌红强硬,为脏腑实热已极。"临床多见于高热惊厥,常见高热、抽搐、神昏、谵语等症状。

内伤病舌强多见于中风(脑血管意外)或中风先兆,中医辨证属风痰阻络者,舌象表现为舌体强硬,舌质较紫暗,舌苔多厚腻。常伴有语言或吞咽不利,口眼歪斜麻木,半身不遂脉弦滑等症状。

【治法】治疗前者清心开窍,后者化痰清腑。

Ⅱ. The Stiff Tongue(Figure 4.1)

A disease referring to the root of the tongue has become stiff. This condition occurs because of attack by exterior evil or internal injury. If exterior heat evil attacks the pericardium in exogenous febrile diseases, it can cause the stagnation of heat and phlegm that block blood vessels, leaving the tongue from getting enough nourishment, manifested as the stiff tongue in crimson color and yellow, sticky or dry coating. So in the book *Bianshe zhi nan* (A Guide to Differentiation of Tongues) it is said:"the red and stiff tongue means the excess heat in Zang-Fu". In clinic the other symptoms consequently seen are high-fever, convulsion, coma, delirium etc.

For the stiffness due to internal injury the main cause is apoplexy (cerebrovascular accident). According to the traditional Chinese medical theory, this condition belongs to wind-phlegm stagnating in the collateral, reflected on the tongue texture as stiffy, dark purple tongue body, and heavy coating. Other symptoms are difficult to speak, facial paralysis, hemiplegia, and taut slippery pulse.

【treatment】For the former treated by removing heart-heat to restore consciousness; for the latter treated by eliminating phlegm and purging bowels.

三、歪斜舌(图 4.2)

伸舌时舌体歪向一侧,称为歪斜舌。此舌象最多见于中风(内风证)或中风后遗症(多属现代医学之脑血管意外,这种舌歪是中枢性面瘫的表现),根据病情轻重,本症状既可单独出现,也可与神志障碍、半身不遂等症状同见,前者病位浅、病情轻,中医学辨证为"中经络",后者病位深、病情重,辨证为"中脏腑"。

除此之外,歪斜舌还可见于舌下神经损伤及周围性面神经麻痹等局部病变,中医辨证多属"外风"证。

Ⅲ. The Deviated Tongue(Figure 4.2)

Deviation of the tongue refers to the tongue aslant to one side of the mouth. This usually happens in apoplexy or its sequel. In modern medicine this is a symptom of cerebrovascular accident. This may be the only sign in the illness, or accompanied by some others, such as coma, hemiparalysis, etc. The former is the mild type of apoplexy and it is termed "apoplexy involving meridians and collateral". The latter is the serious one and it is considered "apoplexy involving Zang-Fu organs". Besides, some other illnesses may also cause deviation of the tongue, such as damage of the nerve on the underside of the tongue or peripheral facial paralysis. For the traditional Chinese medicine, they are the syndrome of "exogenous wind" syndrome.

四、颤动舌

伸舌时,舌体不自主地抖动、震颤,称为舌颤动。舌体颤动是动风的表现，由于肝为风木之脏，主筋，故凡因高热、肝阳亢逆、阴液或气血虚损等原因影响肝所主的筋脉，使筋脉失养，就会出现所谓“风证”，表现为肢体抽搐震颤，筋挛肉瞤，头摇不定，舌体颤动等症状。热极生风证舌象为：舌红绛或紫绛而颤动；阴虚风动舌象见舌红少苔，舌体瘦薄微微抖动；气血两虚者则为舌质淡白而颤动。

【治法】治疗前者宜清肝凉血熄风；中者用滋阴定风；后者宜大补气血。

Ⅳ. The Trembling Tongue

The trembling tongue refers to the tongue shaking when it is protruding. It is a sign of wind symptoms. According to TCM, the liver is an organ corresponding to wind-wood and dominating the tendons. Many reasons, such as high fever, hyperactivity of the liver yang, deficient yin fluid, or insufficiency of Qi and blood, can leave the tendons short of nourishment, giving rise to "the wind symptom". It is manifested as convulsion or spasm of the body and limbs, trembling of the tendons and muscles, shaking of the head and tongue, etc. The tongue for wind symptom due to extreme heat: it is red or crimson and trembling. The tongue for wind symptom caused by yin-deficiency: it is thin, red color, less coating and slightly shaking. For deficiency of both Qi and blood, it shows pale and trembling.

【Treatment】 For extreme heat causing wind: clearing away the liver-heat to cool blood and arrest wind, for wind caused by yin-deficiency: nourishing yin to subdue wind, for wind due to deficiency of both Qi and blood: benefiting both Qi and blood.

五、吐舌、弄舌

吐舌是指舌伸出口外不能立即收回，经常露出口外；弄舌，是指舌微出口外，旋即缩回口中，或舐口唇四周，上下左右，掉动不停。

吐舌和弄舌都属心脾有热，以致筋脉不舒。但在病危时出现吐舌，则多为疫毒攻心或正气衰败，往往全舌青紫,病属危重。此外,吐舌和弄舌都可见于先天愚型患者。

Ⅴ. The Protrusion and Shaking of the Tongue

Protrusion of the tongue means the tongue protruding out of the mouth and it can not draw back easily. Shaking of the tongue refers to the tongue protruding from the mouth and withdrawing immediately, or licking around the lips and trembling.

Both of them are due to the heat in the heart and spleen. At the serious stage, it is caused by heat-toxin attacking the heart or the failure of vital Qi. The whole tongue is blue purple. Besides, both conditions can be seen in congenital idiocy.

六、短缩舌(图 4.3)

舌体短缩,不能伸出,甚至伸舌不能抵齿,称为舌短缩。

如舌短缩,舌淡白或青紫而湿润,多为寒凝筋脉,或气血虚衰,属虚属寒;如舌短缩,舌红绛而干,多为热盛津伤;若舌敛缩如荔枝干肉,完全没有津液,则为肝肾阴竭,属危重舌象;若舌短缩而胖大苔腻,多为风痰阻络,可见于中风证。

先天性舌系带过短,亦可影响舌体的伸出,称为"绊舌",无辨证意义,可通过手术治疗,临证时应注意排除这种情况。

Ⅵ. The Shortened and Retracted Tongue(Figure 4.3)

When the tongue is short or curled and can not protrude even to teeth, it is called the retracted tongue. Cold accumulation in channels or deficiency of Qi and blood can cause a retracted wet tongue in pale or blue color. Excess heat leads to a retracted withered tongue with red and crimson color. Failure of the liver-Yin and kidney-Yin leads to a retracted dry tongue with no fluid, which is a serious condition. The stagnation of wind-phlegm in the channels causes a swollen retracted tongue with greasy coating. This is commonly seen in apoplexy patients.

Some people are born with a congenitally shortened frenulum of the tongue. This can be solved through surgical operations.

第5章 望苔质

苔质，指苔的形质，主要包括舌苔的厚薄、润燥、腐腻、偏全、剥落、消长、有根无根等内容，分述如下：

Chapter 5 Inspection of the Coating Proper

The coating proper refers to appearance and quality of the coating. It can be inspected in different ways, mainly including its thick or thin, moist or dry, curdy or sticky property, exfoliating or full, wane and wax, with root or without root about the coating, etc.

一、厚薄

【舌象】苔质的厚薄是以“见底”或“不见底”作为衡量标准的，凡能透过舌苔而隐隐见到舌质的，称为“见底”，属于薄苔(图5.1)；由于舌苔遮盖而见不到苔下之舌质者，称为“不见底”，属于厚苔(图5.2)。

【机理】正常人舌上有一层薄白苔，在疾病过程中，舌苔的厚薄变化，主要可反映邪正的盛衰，尤其是可反映邪气的轻重。外感疾病初起或内伤杂病轻浅者及处于疾病恢复期的患者，由于邪气不盛或胃气渐复，所以舌苔多正常；如胃之气阴不足影响舌苔的生成，可见舌苔特别薄，似有似无，即所谓“透明苔”，主气虚；如邪气过盛与胃气相抟结上蒸于舌面即可形成厚苔，所以，根据舌苔的厚薄来判断病邪的轻重具有重要的临床意义。临床观察表明，凡舌苔薄者，病情多轻，预后较好；相反，凡舌苔厚者，病情多重。此外，舌苔厚薄的动态变化，还可反映病势的进退，凡舌苔由薄变厚，提示邪气渐盛，为病进；舌苔由厚渐化变薄，提示正气胜邪，为病退。

【主病】薄苔主外感表证或内伤轻病；厚苔主邪气亢盛，主里证。

【治法】解表;清里。

Ⅰ. Thick or Thin Coating

【Manifestations】The thin or thick coating is judged by whether it can reveal the tongue texture or not. If the tongue texture can be seen vaguely through the coating, it is regarded as the thin coating(Figure 5.1); otherwise it is considered the thick one(Figure 5.2).

【Mechanism】The tongue of a healthy person manifests as a layer of thin white coating. In the process of illness, the thick or thin coating mainly reflects excess or decline of vital Qi and pathogens, especially the condition of pathogens. In the initial stage of the exogenous disease, or mild cases of the internal injury, or recovery period of illness, the coating is mostly normal because of pathogens weakened and the stomach Qi restored gradually. If the stomach Qi and yin is insufficient, the formation of the coating will be affected, and the very thin coating can occur, as if no one, known as "the transparent coating", suggesting Qi deficiency. If pathogen is over excess, it can mix with the stomach Qi, steamed upwards to the tongue, forming the thick coating. Thereby the thick coating is of importance in judging serious degree of pathogens. By clinical observation, it is shown that almost all the thin coating indicates mild illnesses with favorable prognosis, and contrarily the thick one means severe diseases. Moreover, the developing change between thick and thin coating can reflect advance or retreat of pathological condition. If the coating changes from thin to thick one, it means, pathogens become excess and disease is worse. Otherwise it denotes vital Qi acts upon pathogens and disease is better.

【Indication】The thin coating indicates the exterior syndrome or the mild cases of the internal injury; The thick coating suggests pathogen excess and the interior syndrome.

【Treatment】To relieve the exterior, or to purge the interior.

二、润、燥、糙、滑

【舌象】舌面润泽，干湿适中为“润苔”（参见图5.1）；舌面水分过多，望之水滑，甚则伸舌欲滴，扪之湿而滑，称为“滑苔”（图5.3）或“水滑苔”；望之干燥，扪之无津，是为“燥苔”，严重者颗粒粗糙干裂如砂石，扪之糙手，称为“糙苔”（图5.4）。

【机理及主病】望舌苔的润燥，主要可了解津液的盈亏及其输布情况。润苔是正常舌苔的表现之一，在疾病中见到润苔，说明津液未伤，津液在体内的代谢基本正常，各种对津液无损伤的疾病（如风寒表证、内伤病轻证）均可见润苔。滑苔则主寒湿重证，为水寒内聚之象，多因三焦阳气衰少，不能温化水液，导致湿停水聚，水湿上泛于舌，即见舌苔水滑，临证常见于肺、脾、肾阳虚而水湿痰饮内停者。

燥苔的辨证意义有两点，其一是提示体内津液已伤，这是燥苔形成的主要原因，多见于感受温燥邪气、高热、大汗、吐泻、饮水不足或过服温燥药物等，致使体内水分丧失过多，津液不足，舌苔失于濡润而现干燥之象。

其二是人体的阳气被阴邪（如痰饮、水湿之类）所遏阻，不能蒸化津液以濡润舌苔，故可见到所谓“腻干苔”，属津液气化及输布障碍。

糙苔多由燥苔进一步发展而成，舌苔干结粗糙，津液全无，多见于热盛伤阴的重证。若苔质粗糙而不干者，多为秽浊盘踞中焦脾胃。临证应注意二者的鉴别，前者治疗在于滋阴补液，后者则宜祛除胃中秽浊。

【治法】白滑苔：外感寒湿宜辛温解表；内伤脾肾阳虚宜温中渗湿。黄滑苔：治宜渗利湿热。燥苔、糙苔用清热生津。

Ⅱ. The Moist, Dry, Rough, and Watery Coating

【Manifestations】The surface of a tongue shows moist with moderate fluid termed the moist coating(see Figure 5.1), while the surface of the tongue appears excessive fluid and looks watery, even ready to drip when protruding the tongue, feeling wet and smooth, known as watery coating(Figure 5.3). Otherwise, looking dry and feeling no fluid, it is the "the dry coating". In the severe case, the coating with its grains as rough and dry as sands, feeling unsmoothed, is called "the rough coating" (Figure 5.4).

【Mechanism and Indications】 Observation of moist and dry tongue is used to learn the conditions of wax or wane as well as distribution of the body fluids. The moist coating is one of normal signs of the tongue. If occurring in diseases, it means the body fluid unimpaired, and water metabolism under normal condition. Usually it is seen in such diseases as the exterior syndrome due to wind-cold, or mild syndrome of the internal injury, which can not cause consumption of the body fluid.

The watery coating suggests severe syndrome of dampness-cold, being a sign of accumulation of water cold in the interior. It is formed by upward floating of water-dampness that is stagnation due to deficient Yang of the triple-Jiao and its poor warming transformation for water fluid. Clinically this coating is usually seen in cases of water dampness or phlegm retention caused by insufficient Yang of the lung, spleen and kidney.

The dry coating has two kinds of significance in syndrome differentiation. Firstly, it denotes injury of the body fluid, which is the main reason for dry coating formation. It is usually seen in the sufferer of exogenous warm or dry pathogen, or in cases of high fever, profuse sweating, vomiting, diarrhea, shortness of drinking, and over intake of warm-dry medications, etc. For the body fluid can be consumed under such conditions, it is not sufficient to moisten the tongue coating, bringing a dry sign.

Secondly, it results from obstruction of Yang Qi by yin evils, such as phlegm fluid, and water dampness, etc. The body fluid fails to be transformed and distributed to the tongue, leading to "the sticky and dry coating", attributable to disorder of fluid distribution.

The rough coating is usually a further development of the dry one. It is characterized by dry, hard and rough appearance without any fluid at all, usually seen in the severe case of yin exhaustion by extreme heat. In another hand, if the texture of coating is rough but no any dry sign, it indicates turbidity remaining in the spleen and stomach of the middle-Jiao. In the clinic practice, attention should be paid to distinguish these two types. The former can be treated by nourishing yin fluid, and the latter by expelling turbidity from the stomach.

【Treatment】 To the white watery coating: If affected by exogenous cold dampness, the treatment should be relieving the exterior syndrome with acrid and warm medicine. If seen in the internal injury case of the spleen and kidney Yang deficiency, it should be treated by warming the middle and excreting dampness. To the yellow watery coating: The method of clearing away heat and excreting dampness should be adopted. To the dried coating or rough coating: The treatment is to clear away heat and produce body fluid.

三、腐腻

【舌象】苔质颗粒粗大，质地疏松，形如豆腐渣厚积于舌面，揩之可去，称为“腐苔”（图 5.5）。舌质颗粒细腻致密，融合成片，中心较厚，紧贴于舌面，揩之不去，刮之不脱，称为“腻苔”（图 5.6）。因形态略具差异，腻苔还可再细分为若干种，如苔腻而垢浊的，称为“垢腻苔”；腻苔上罩有一层稠厚粘液的，称为“粘腻苔”；苔腻湿润水滑的，称为“滑腻苔”；苔腻干燥少津的，称为“腻干苔”，但无论何种腻苔，均以苔质细腻板滞，不易脱落为特征。

【机理及主病】腐苔多为阳热有余，蒸发胃中腐浊邪气上升于舌而成，主要见于食积痰浊或内痈等病证。一般病程中，舌苔由板滞不宣而化腐，由腐而退，渐生浮薄新苔，是正气胜邪，病邪解尽之象。

腻苔多由湿浊内蕴，阳气被其阻遏所致，其主病为湿浊、痰饮、食积不化等。苔白滑腻为湿从寒化，病因为外感湿邪并内伤脾虚湿重。如湿邪化热，湿热交阻出现黄腻苔。若腻苔与厚苔并见，标志邪气较盛；厚腻苔持续不退，则往往表示病情加重、恶化或迁延难愈。

【治法】腐苔多为邪热有余，治宜祛除有余邪热。腻苔每属阳气被抑，治疗尚需结合苔色而定，一般而言，白腻苔宜芳香化浊，温中燥湿；黄腻苔宜清热化湿（可参见第8章内容）。

Ⅲ. The Curdy and Sticky Coating

【Manifestations】Curdy Coating (Figure 5.5): The coating grains are rough, big and loose, as if a heap of soy bean curd dregs thickly remaining on the tongue surface easily to be scraped off.

Sticky Coating(Figure 5.6): The coating grains are fine, dense and integrated, showing thick on the tongue center, sticking to the tongue surface hard to be scrubbed off. The sticky coating can be subdivided into four types according to different appearances. (1) The sticky coating with turbidity is named "the turbid-sticky coating". (2) The sticky coating with a layer of thick mucus is termed "the sticky coating". (3) The sticky coating showing moist and watery is defined as "the slippery-sticky coating". (4) The sticky coating marked by dry or less fluid is described as "the sticky-dry coating". All the sticky coatings are characterized by fine and sticky appearance, and hard to go off.

【Mechanism and Indications】The curdy fur is formed due to excessive yang heat, which steams the rotten turbid Qi of the stomach up to the tongue and forms the coating. It is mainly seen in cases of accumulation of indigested food, or phlegm turbidity, and internal abscess. In the general course of diseases, if the fur is changing from sticky, dense to loose and curdy, from curdy to decrease, instead, gradually growing the new and thin coating, it is a sign of vital Qi acting upon pathogens that have been eliminated.

The sticky fur results mainly from accumulation of turbid dampness in the interior as well as blockage of yang Qi by it. The indications of the coating are stagnant dampness turbidity, phlegm fluid, and indigested food. Thc white sticky coating indicates dampness pathogen transformed into cold, the etiology for that is invasion of exogenous pathogenic dampness, complicated with endogenous dampness due to the spleen deficiency in the internal injury. The yellow sticky coating suggests dampness pathogen transformed into heat, damp heat mixing together and obstructing the interior. When the sticky coating shows thick, it denotes the pathogen is intense. The thick and sticky coating lasts a long period without any improvement, usually implying the disease worsened, or lingering and hard to recover.

【Treatment】For the curdy fur means pathogenic heat excessive, the treatment should aim at eliminating excessive heat pathogen. For the sticky fur suggests obstruction of Yang Qi, the therapy should be made according to the color of the tongue. Generally speaking, the white and sticky coating should be treated as eliminating dampness with either fragrant medicine or bitter-warm herbs. The yellow and sticky coating should be clearing away heat and resolving dampness.

四、偏全

【舌象】舌苔满布舌面称为“全”(图 5.7)。舌苔半布,偏于前(外)、后(内)、左、右某一局部者,称为“偏”。本照片厚苔偏中后(图 5.8)。

【机理及主病】舌苔的偏全,是言舌苔的分布情况。察舌苔分布的偏全,可以诊察病变之所在。正常舌苔应为薄而均匀,以中根部稍厚,全苔主邪气弥漫,多为湿痰阻滞中焦之象。若中根部的苔过于厚腻,则说明脾有痰湿,胃肠积滞。舌苔偏于左右一侧,为邪在半表半里;因舌边属肝胆,所以也见于肝胆病变。

Ⅳ. The Full Coating or Partial Coating

【Manifestations】The coating is fully distributed on the surface of the tongue termed “the full coating”(Figure 5.7), while it is half distributed at the front tongue, back tongue, or left, right side of the tongue, regarded as “the partial coating”. The tongue on the picture shows a thick coating partly at the center and back(Figure 5.8).

【Mechanism and Indications】The coating of full or half

depicts conditions of the coating distribution. Observation of the coating distribution can learn the location of the disease. The normal coating should be thin and even, only with the slight thick middle and root parts. The full coating indicates pathogenic factors filling the body, and it is a sign of obstruction of the middle-Jiao by dampness phlegm. If the coating is over thick at the middle and root tongue, it indicates phlegm dampness in the spleen as well as indigested food in the stomach and intestines. The half coating on the left or right suggests pathogen located between the exterior and interior, or disorders of the liver and gallbladder, since the sides of the tongue are related to the liver-gallbladder.

五、剥落

【舌象】舌苔部分脱落,脱落处光滑无苔,称为“剥苔”或“花剥苔”(图5.9)。舌苔大片剥落,边缘凸起,界限清楚剥脱部位不固定,时时转移者,称为“地图舌”(图5.10),也属剥苔,是剥苔的一种类型。如舌面剥苔处不光滑,仍有新生的薄苔颗粒可见,称为“类剥苔”(图5.11)。若舌苔全部剥落殆尽,舌面无苔,光滑如同镜面者,称为“镜面舌”(图5.12),是剥苔中最严重的一种。

【机理及主病】观苔之剥落,可测胃气、胃阴之存亡,推断疾病的预后。舌苔是由胃气上蒸脾湿而成,是脾胃功能健全的标志,若久病、重病导致胃气、胃阴不足,或气血两虚,不能上承以续生新苔,舌苔即可出现剥落,其中尤以阴虚舌红苔剥最为常见。若花剥而兼有厚腻苔,多为痰浊邪气未化而正气已伤,病情更为严重。舌质淡而有花剥苔,多为血虚或气血两虚。类剥苔常见于久病之后,舌苔曾一度出现剥落,由于正气渐复,又新生出薄苔,主病久气血不续。

“镜面舌”是剥苔中最严重的一种,多见于重病阶段,提示胃阴干涸、胃气大伤,胃已毫无生发之气,完全不能上潮以成苔,故舌面光洁如镜。临证见镜面舌,不论其色为何,皆属胃气将绝的危候,若淡白而光莹,是脾胃损伤,气血亏损已极;若红绛而光剥,是水涸火炎,胃阴枯竭之兆。

Ⅴ. The Exfoliative Fur

【Manifestations】 The tongue coating peeled off partially is known as "the exfoliated coating"(Figure 5.9), or "the scattered exfoliative coating". If the coating is exfoliated mostly with the border raised and obvious, and the site is unfixed to move frequently, it is named "the map tongue"(Figure 5.10), belonging to one type of exfoliative coating. In another condition, the peeled region is not smooth, showing some thin grains of coating newly growing, which is described as "the exfoliative kind of coating"(Figure 5.11). If the coating peels off completely and the tongue is as smooth and glossy as a mirror, it is termed "the mirror-like tongue" that is the most serious one among the exfoliative coating(Figure 5.12).

【Mechanism and Indications】 By observing the exfoliation of the coating, the existence or exhaustion of the stomach Qi and yin may be learned, and prognosis of illness can be made. For the coating of the tongue is formed as a result of upward steaming of the stomach Qi upon the spleen yin. So it becomes the sign of the normal function of the spleen and stomach. If prolonged and severe diseases cause the stomach Qi or yin insufficient, or deficiency of Qi and blood, the tongue will be failure in nourishment and in growing the new coating, then exfoliative coating occurs consequently. Among the exfoliative coatings, the red tongue due to yin deficiency accompanied with the peeled coating is mostly seen clinically. If the exfoliated coating together with sticky and thick coating, it means retention of turbid phlegm complicated with impairment of vital Qi, suggesting more severity of pathological condition. The pale tongue with exfoliated coating is usually formed due to insufficient blood or both blood and Qi deficiency. The exfoliation-like coating often occurs after prolonged diseases, because the tongue coating once peeled in process of illness and newly developed while vital Qi restoring gradually, indicating less supply of Qi and blood in prolonged diseases.

The mirror-like tongue is the most serious one among the exfoliated coatings. It is usually seen at the severe stage of diseases, resulting from exhaustion of both the stomach yin and the stomach Qi. The stomach has no vitality at all and loses the ability for supplying upwards and generating the coating on the tongue, so the tongue shows as glossy as a mirror. If the mirror-like tongue occurs clinically, no matter what color with it, all belong to a dangerous sign of the stomach Qi disappearance. Among them, the pale tongue showing glossy is the result of extreme deficiency of the Qi and blood due to impairment of the spleen and stomach, but the red crimson tongue with exfoliated coating is caused by stomach yin exhaustion and the internal fire hyperactivity.

六、消长

【舌象】"消",是舌苔由厚变薄、由多变少地消退;"长",是舌苔由无而有,由薄变厚地增长。

【机理及主病】舌苔的消长变化,反映着邪正相争的过程,据此可以判断疾病的进退吉凶。凡舌苔由少变多、由薄变厚,一般来讲说明邪气渐盛,主病进;反之,舌苔由厚变薄、由多变少,则说明正胜邪退,主病退。但无论是消还是长,都以渐变为佳,即应有一个渐消渐长的过程,若骤长骤消、骤增骤退,多为病情暴变的征象,如薄苔突然增厚,说明正气暴衰,邪气急剧入里;若满舌厚苔骤然消退,往往是胃气暴绝的反映。

Ⅵ. Wane and Wax of the Tongue Coating

【Manifestations】"Wane" refers to change of the coating from thick to thin, or from much to less, while "wax" refers to increasing of the coating from absence to appearance, from thin to thick.

【Mechanism and Indications】Wane and wax of the tongue coating reflect a process of struggling between vital Qi and pathogens. Accordingly the improvement or aggravation of illness can be judged. If the coating grows, it indicates pathogen tuning excessively and disease advanced. In the contrary, it means the vital Qi recovery with pathogen retreat, suggesting improvement of diseases. It will be better that the wane or wax of coating changes gradually. It is a worse sign if the thickness of coating varies suddenly, meaning an abrupt advance of diseases. For example, the thin coating turns to thick swiftly, showing a fast decline of vital Qi and a rapid invasion of the interior by pathogen. But the full and thick coating disappears quickly, reflecting critical exhaustion of the stomach Qi.

七、有根、无根

【舌象】临证观舌,凡舌苔坚敛着实,紧贴舌面,刮之难去,像从舌体长出来,即为“有根苔”,又称“真苔”;若苔不着实,似浮涂舌上,刮之即去,不像是从舌上生出来的,称为“无根苔”,又叫“假苔”。图 5.13 为无根假苔,图 5.14 为无根浮垢苔。

【机理及主病】观舌之有根、无根,有极重要的临床意义:有根之苔,是脾胃生发之气熏蒸上聚于舌而成的,故凡有根苔无论厚薄,均提示正气未衰。其中有根之薄苔,匀铺于舌面之上,苔质比较疏松活泛,属正常苔,是胃气旺盛的表现,见于正常健康人或有表证、轻病的患者,提示正气充足,邪气轻微;有根的厚苔,虽表示邪气较盛,但正气尚充,脾胃之气与邪气抟结上潮于舌而成厚苔,故多见于实证。而无根之苔则不然。无根苔无论厚薄,均标志机体正气衰竭。尤多见于胃、脾、肾之气阴大伤。故见无根之苔必为虚证。为了更加准确地判断舌苔有根无根,临证应注意使用揩舌、刮舌法。

Ⅶ. The Tongue Coating with Root or without any Root

【Manifestations】 If the tongue is covered with densely smooth coating that sticks to the tongue and hard to scrape off, as if growing from the tongue body, it is termed “the root coating”, or “the real coating”. While the tongue is with loosely scattered coating and easy to scrub off, as if not growing from the tongue, is described as “the coating without any root”, or “the false coating”. The figure 5.13 are false fur without any root. And the figure 5.14 are the loosely dirty fur without any root.

【Mechanism and Indications】 Observation of the coating with a root or without any root is great importance in clinic. Since the coating with root is produced by upward steaming of the spleen and stomach vital Qi. The coating with root, no matter it is thin or thick, denotes vital Qi under sufficient condition without decline. The thin coating with a root distributed evenly shows loose and lively, belonging to the normal coating, as a manifestation of abundant stomach Qi. It is often seen in a healthy person, or the exterior syndrome, or the mild cases. It suggests sufficient vital Qi and slight pathogen. But the thick coating with a root indicates pathogen excessive and vital Qi sufficient as well. It is formed as a result of upward steaming of the spleen and stomach Qi in combination with pathogens, often found in excess syndromes. It is not the same as the coating without any root. If the coating is without any root, it typifies the failure of vital Qi, no matter thin or thick it is, frequently seen in deficient syndromes, caused by severe damage of both Qi and yin within the stomach, spleen, and kidney. In order to distinguish these two types of fur exactly, scrub and scrape methods should be tried clinically.

第6章 望苔色

舌苔的颜色，简称苔色。主病的苔色，主要有白、黄、灰、黑四种，在疾病发展过程中，还可见兼色，如黄白苔、灰黑苔等。古代医家在长期的医疗实践中逐渐发现，不同性质的邪气所致的病证反映于舌，会出现不同颜色的苔，而且随着病证的变化，苔色也会发生相应的改变，如白苔者，病在表；黄苔者，病在里；灰黑苔，病在肾。苔色由白而黄，由黄而黑者，病日进；苔色由黑而黄，由黄而白者，病日退。由此可见，辨苔色主要用于辨别病邪的性质和推断病情的轻重进退。

Chapter 6 Inspection of the Coating Color

The color of the tongue fur is termed coating color. Coating colors related to diseases have four classes, including white, yellow, gray and black. During a process of illness, two colors of coating can be seen simultaneously, such as white-yellow fur, black-gray fur, etc. Through long period of clinical practice, ancient doctors found that the coating color can reflect different problems caused by different evil Qi, and it may also change along with the pathological conditions. For example, the white coating means the exterior syndrome, while the yellow coating means the interior syndrome, and the black-gray coating reflects the kidney disease. So when the coating color turns from white to yellow or from yellow to black, it means the disease advanced. But if it changes from black to yellow or from yellow to white, it marks the better of illness. Therefore, through the coating color we can learn the nature and depth of diseases.

一、白苔

白苔是临床最为常见的苔色，其他各种苔色皆由此转化而成。一般多见于表证和寒证。白苔主表，是由于外感邪气尚未传里，里热未起，舌苔往往还未发生明显的变化，仍为正常时的薄白苔，白苔除主表外，也多见于寒证或寒湿证，《辨舌指南》说："寒湿本阴邪，白为凉象。"故无论是实寒证还是虚寒证，均以白苔为其基本苔色。但需注意的是，寒证、寒湿证所形成的白苔往往比较湿润粘滑厚腻，与表证或正常人的薄白清爽之苔有所不同，临证应注意这些差别。

在某些特殊情况下，白苔也可见于热证，为白苔主病之变。如舌上满布白苔，似白粉堆积，扪之不燥，称为"积粉苔"，其形成是由于外感秽浊不正之气，毒热内盛所致，常见于瘟疫（一些急性烈性传染病）或内痈（内脏的化脓性感染）。再如苔白糙裂如砂石，扪之粗糙干涩，称为"糙裂苔"或"白砂苔"，这种白苔也主热证，其形成机理主要是由于温热邪气太盛，邪热化燥入里迅速，以致苔色还未来得及转黄，津液已经大伤，也为白苔中的一个特殊类型。这些特殊的白苔提示我们，白苔的辨证不可教条地局限于主表主寒，而应注意结合舌质、苔质的变化，以及其他诊法所获得的资料综合起来加以分析，才不致有误。

临床观察认为，白苔除可见于正常人外，多见于疾病初起、疾病的恢复期和一些相对来讲较轻微的病证，故凡舌见白苔，特别是薄白苔，一般表示病情不太严重，预后较好，与后面所要论及的黄苔、灰黑苔有显著的不同。

临床常见白苔及主病如下。

Ⅰ. The White Tongue Coating

This is a kind of coating condition commonly seen in clinic. Other colors of coating are developed from it. Usually the white coating indicates the exterior syndrome as well as cold syndrome. For the former, the exogenous evils haven't transmitted into the interior and the interior heat has not occurred, leaving the coating color unaffected, which is still as usual as white. For the latter, it is explained in an ancient book named *Bian She Zhi Nan* (A Guide to Differentiation of the Tongue) that "Pathogenic cold and wet belong to Yin evils, and white color is the manifestation of cold Yin". For this reason, no matter excess cold or deficiency cold, the white of coating is the basic color. But with cold nature, the coating is marked by moisture, greasy and thickness, which is different from the thin coating of the exterior syndrome or normal people. This should be paid more attention to in clinical diagnosis.

On the other hand, the white coating may also be seen in some heat cases. Under such conditions, the coating appears white thick and full, as if it was heaped by white powder, but it is not dry when felt. This is called "powder coating". The reason for that is heat-toxin excess in the interior, which is developed from exogenous turbid evil affected by the body. This is commonly seen in infectious epidemic disease (acute infectious disease), or abscess of internal organs (pyogenic infection of internal organs). In the other case, the white coating looks drying like rough sand called "white sand coating" or "rough coating". The result of it is extremely excessive heat, which impairs body fluid and transmits into the interior too fast to bring the tongue into yellow color, leaving the tongue still as white. All these unusual manifestation show that white coating reflects not only the exterior and cold syndromes but also other heat syndromes. So it is necessary to analyze all signs and comprehend different methods to make the final diagnosis.

In addition, it is usually considered that the white coating of tongue indicates the onset of illness, restoration stage, as well as some mild illnesses. So the white coating, especially thin and white coating means that the disease is not critical and has a favorite prognosis. This is different from the yellow, gray, or black coating obviously that will be discussed latter.

The white coatings commonly seen and their indications are as follows.

1. **薄白苔(图6.1)**

【舌象】苔色白,苔质薄而清爽干净,薄薄地平铺于舌面上,其下舌质的颜色仍可透出而不被完全遮盖,中部已略见增厚,干润适中。在外感表证中,由于所感邪气性质不同,故在薄白苔的基础上可略有差异,外感风寒证苔薄白而润，舌色如常或略淡；外感风热表证舌苔薄白略干，舌边尖红；外感寒湿表证，苔薄白而滑，舌质较暗淡。

【主病】表证；轻证。薄白苔为正常舌苔的表现，也可见于外感表证初起或各种内伤杂病病情轻浅无明显热象者。中医学认为，舌苔的形成是由胃中生气所现。正常人胃气充盛且无邪气，故苔质苔色即现正常，病轻之人或表证初起，邪气均较轻微，对胃气的干扰或损伤十分轻浅，所以舌苔仍能保持在正常状态。

【治法】解表；对证治疗。

1. The Thin and White Coating(Figure 6.1)

【Manifestations】A white, thin and moss-like layer is distributed evenly on the surface of tongue. Through the layer the tongue property can be vaguely seen. Ifaffected by exogenous wind-cold, the coating is thin, white and moisture, and the color of tongue property is still as normal or light pale. If affected by exogenous wind-heat, the coating is thin, white and slightly dry, with the color of tongue edges and tip red. If affected by exogenous wet-cold, the coating is thin, white and watery, and the color of tongue property is dim pale.

【Indications】The exterior syndrome, or mild cases. Usually the thin and white coating of tongue is a normal manifestation. Besides that, it can also occur in the exterior disease or various internal injury diseases that have no obvious heat sign. According to traditional Chinese medical theory, the coating of tongue is formed as a result of the stomach Qi. In normal people, the tongue coating results from the ordinary stomach Qi without evils. When in disease, the evil Qi is mild at the beginning stage and it can not make disturbance or any damage to the stomach Qi, so the coating of tongue can be kept as usual.

【Treatment】To relieve the exterior syndrome, or to give expectant treatment.

2. **白厚苔(图6.2)**

【舌象】苔色白，苔质较厚，甚至不能“见底”(即不能看到下面的舌质色)。

【主病】风寒邪盛；中焦寒湿邪盛。白厚苔是邪气盛的表现。外感病若见到舌苔由薄白渐变为白厚,由较浮松变为紧贴舌面刮而不脱,说明风寒邪气较盛,寒邪有化火入里的趋势。内伤杂病见此舌苔,也说明寒、湿、痰、食等邪气内盛,如舌质色正常或较红,表明正气尚盛,能够抗邪;若舌质淡白而见白厚苔者提示正虚邪盛,是邪气胜正的表现。

【治法】辛温散寒;温中燥湿。

2. The Thick and White Coating(Figure 6.2)

【Manifestations】 The coating is thick and white. The tongue proper can not be observed clearly through the coating.

【Indications】 Excessive pathogenic wind cold or cold dampness retention in the middle-Jiao. Thick and white coating is the symptom of excessive evil Qi. If in exogenous disease, the white coating changes from thin to thick, from loose to dense attaching to the tongue hard to scrape off, suggesting pathogenic cold-wind hyperactive with a tendency transforming into heat and attacking the interior. If in internal injury diseases it means pathogens are excess, such as cold, dampness, phlegm, and indigested food. When this type of coating is present with a normal tongue or red tongue, it suggests the vital Qi strong enough to struggle against the evil Qi. If it appears with the pale tongue, it denotes the evil Qi hyperactivity over the vital Qi.

【Treatment】 To dispel cold with warm and pungent medicine, or to warm the middle-Jiao for eliminating dampness.

3. **白滑苔**(图6.3)

【舌象】苔白水滑,甚则张口伸舌欲滴,舌涎清冷,舌质淡白胖嫩。

【主病】脾肾阳虚,水饮内停。此舌象主要见于里虚寒证,特别是脾肾阳虚。脾肾两脏与人体水液代谢关系最为密切,脾主运化水液,"肾者水脏,主津液",人体水液代谢的正常进行主要依赖于脾肾二脏阳气的充足,若脾肾二脏阳气不足,对水液的温煦气化作用必然减退,水液不能蒸腾气化升清降浊,就会变成痰饮水湿等病理产物停聚体内,水气上溢即可见舌苔湿润水滑、舌体胖大。临床常见有面白肢冷,眼睑浮肿,倦怠嗜睡,水肿尿少,肠鸣泄泻,涕唾痰涎稀薄清冷等水寒内停的症状。

外感寒湿证也可出现白滑苔,属寒湿实证,故无虚损之象,舌质一般也不会出现胖大白嫩,不难鉴别。

【治法】温阳利水。

3. The Watery and White Coating(Figure 6.3)

【Manifestations】The coating is white and watery, seen much thin cold saliva tending to drop. The tongue proper is pale, enlarged, and tender.

【Indications】The spleen and kidney Yang deficiency with water dampness retention. This is mostly caused by the deficiency of both spleen-Yang and kidney-Yang. The spleen and kidney have close relation with water metabolism. The spleen can transport and transform the water fluid while the kidney can regulates the whole activity of water metabolism. So insufficient Yang in the spleen and kidney will result in accumulation of the phlegm dampness, which float upward to the tongue and bring it watery and enlarged. Many symptoms linked with the tongue can occur, such as pale complexion, cold extremities, swollen eyelid, lassitude, lethargy, edema, diarrhea, oliguria, clear saliva, etc.

In addition, this type of coating can be caused by exogenous cold dampness too, which belongs to excessive syndrome. But the tongue shows no deficient sign as puffy and tender. So it is easy to identify.

【Treatment】It should be treated by the method of warming Yang to diuresis.

4. **白腻苔(图 6.4)**

【舌象】苔色白,苔质颗粒细腻致密,粘连成片紧贴于舌面,刮之不易脱落。图 6.4 所示的白腻苔已微微发黄,呈双黄苔。

【主病】外感湿邪;湿浊内生。中医病因学认为"湿性粘滞",故凡见到舌苔粘腻不爽,垢浊不清,说明体内有湿邪停着。湿邪的形成既可由于外感,也可由于内生。湿为阴邪,易阻遏气机,损伤阳气,故舌淡苔白腻正是湿邪内停,阳气被其所遏不能伸展之象。

【治法】化湿醒脾;健脾利湿。

4. The White Greasy Coating(Figure 6.4)

【Manifestations】The color of coating is white, dense and sticking tightly on the surface of tongue, so it is difficult to scrape off. Figure 6.4 shows the white greasy coating with some yellowish color. It is termed the double yellow coating.

【Indications】Affection by exogenous dampness, or retention of turbid dampness in the interior. In TCM opinion, "dampness is sticky and stagnant in nature", therefore the dampness-evil is stagnating in the body when finding the greasy and grimy coating. The formation of pathogenic dampness is related to both exogenous and endogenous reasons. Since dampness belongs to the Yin-evil it is easy to obstruct activity of Qi, then Yang involved. Thus the pale and white greasy coating manifests depression of Yang by dampness retention.

【Treatment】To recuperate spleen through dispelling dampness, or to invigorate spleen for eliminating dampness.

5. 白腻干苔(图 6.5)

【舌象】与白腻苔大致相同,边薄中厚,但比较干燥。

【主病】湿阻津承。这种舌苔的形成主要是由于湿浊痰饮停聚于体内,湿浊痰饮作为有形的实邪可阻碍津液的输布,使之不能上承于口,加之脾阳虚损,气化生津的能力也不足,即所谓"生湿不生津",故口舌不得津液的濡润,而见干燥之象,出现白腻干苔。

【治法】扶阳益气,化湿生津。

5. The Dry and White Greasy Coating(Figure 6.5)

【Manifestations】It is similar to the white greasy coating, only dry.

【Indications】Obstruction of the body fluid by dampness. The reasons for the tongue coating are mainly stagnation of dampness turbidity and phlegm. Since dampness phlegm is excessive pathogen, it can retard distribution of the body fluid, and consequently cause the failure of fluid upward to the tongue. The tongue will be short of nourishment, and then the dry sign emerged.

【Treatment】To promote the production of fluid and eliminate the dampness, or to benefit Qi and tonify Yang.

6. 白糙、裂苔(白砂苔)(图 6.6)

【舌象】舌苔白厚干燥粗糙如砂皮,颗粒较大,扪之碍手,无细滑感,舌质红。

【主病】温邪过重,暴热伤津。邪热太盛,入里迅速,苔尚未及转黄而里热已炽,津液暴伤,故见舌红,苔白干燥如砂石。

【治法】急下存阴,泻热生津。

6. The White Tough and Split Coating (white sand coating)(Figure 6.6)

【Manifestations】The coating is white thickness, dry, and rough. It feels like sand. The color of tongue proper is red.

【Indications】Consumption of the body fluid by extremely pathogenic warm heat. The heat-evil is so hyperactive that it invades the interior fast with the coating color unchanged. Owing to excess of heat, the body fluid is consumed seriously. So the tongue gets red and covered with dry, white, and fissured coating like sands.

【Treatment】To purge the bowels urgently for saving fluid, or to expel heat and promote production of the body fluid.

7. 白如积粉苔(图 6.7)

【舌象】舌上满布白苔中见双黄,厚腻如白粉堆积,扪之不燥,舌质略红。

【主病】瘟疫时行之病。这种舌象属白腻苔类,常见于外感温热病,多因外感秽浊不正之气,热毒内盛,夹有湿邪所致。

【治法】清瘟泄热。

7. The White Powder Coating(Figure 6.7)

【Manifestations】The tongue is fully covered by white thickness and greasy coating as if the heap of white powder. It feels no dryness. Within the white coating the yellow color appears (double yellow coating). The tongue body is relatively red.

【Indications】Infection of epidemic disease. The picture

belongs to the type of white greasy coating. It usually occurs in the epidemic febrile disease caused by exogenous evil-Qi combined with wet-evil.

【Treatment】To clear way epidemic febrile.

8. 雪花苔

【舌象】舌苔白如雪花，积于舌面，舌质淡白。

【主病】脾阳衰败，脾冷而闭。这种苔是脾阳竭绝的反映，属危重舌象。由于脾阳衰微，寒湿凝滞中焦，所以出现比一般脾阳虚的白苔更严重的雪花苔。

【治法】温暖脾阳。

8. The Snow Coating

【Manifestations】The white coating seems snow accumulated on the surface of tongue. The tongue proper is pale.

【Indications】Decline of the spleen Yang and obstruction of spleen by cold. This picture reflects exhaustion of the spleen-Yang, which belongs to critical state of disease. Because of the spleen Yang decline, cold dampness stagnates in the middle-Jiao, thus giving rise to the sign of coating like snow.

【Treatment】To warm the spleen-Yang.

二、黄苔

黄苔为外邪入里化热，热邪熏灼所致，故黄苔主里证、热证。在外感病中，舌苔由白转黄，提示邪已入里化热，黄色越深，表示热邪越甚。黄苔多与红、绛舌同见。

黄苔主里证、热证为其主病之常，但在某些情况下，黄苔也可见于表证和虚寒证，如风热、暑、燥诸邪在表，都可出现薄黄苔。阳虚寒湿、痰饮等停滞，郁久化热也可见到黄滑苔，这些情况，都是临证时应当加以注意的。

此外，传统中医学还认为，脾胃病变多见黄苔，“舌为脾之外候”，“苔乃胃气之熏蒸”，脾胃位于中焦，在五行属土，在五色配黄，故脾胃之本色即为黄色。脾胃病变，大多为现代医学的消化系统疾病，如胃炎、肠炎、肝炎、胆囊炎等。

临床常见黄苔及主病如下。

Ⅱ. The Yellow Coating

The yellow coating results from pathogenic heat transformed from exogenous evil, so it indicates the interior syndrome as well as heat syndrome. If in an exterior disease, the color of coating changes from white to yellow, it means that exogenous pathogen has been in the interior and turned into heat nature. The deeper the yellow color, the worse the pathogenic heat. Red or dark purple tongue proper often occurs together with the yellow coating.

In addition, the yellow coating may be seen in the exterior syndrome and deficiency cold syndrome under some conditions. For instance, the exogenous wind-heat, or summer-heat, or dry pathogen can all cause the thin yellow coating when they invade the exterior of body. Moreover a prolonged retention of cold dampness or phlegm due to the deficiency of Yang can transform into heat, leading to the yellow coating. All these should be paid attention to while making diagnosis.

On the other hand, the yellow coating may appear in the spleen and stomach diseases according to TCM theory, for both organs situate in the middle-Jiao, which correspond to the earth and yellow color in the Five Elements Doctrine. While the spleen and stomach have problems, the digestive system will be disorder, such as gastritis, enteronitis, cholecystitis etc.

Yellow coatings commonly seen and their indications are as follows.

1. **薄黄苔**(图 6.8)

【舌象】舌苔在薄白基础上带有浅黄色。

【主病】风热表证;风寒化热未甚。舌苔薄黄提示邪热未甚,多见于风热表证或风寒化热入里,里热尚不甚之证。

【治法】有表证者仍当解表,表证已罢,舌苔纯黄无白才宜清里。

1. The Thin and Yellow Coating(Figure 6.8)

【Manifestations】On the white and thin coating of tongue there is slight yellow color.

【Indications】The exterior syndrome of wind heat, or mild

heat syndrome of the interior transformed from exogenous wind cold. This kind of tongue coating reflects that the heat-evil is not severe. It is mostly seen in the exterior syndrome of wind-heat, or at the beginning stage of internal heat transformed from exogenous wind cold.

【Treatment】To relieve the exterior syndrome, or to eliminate the interior heat.

2. **黄厚(燥)苔**(图 6.9)

【舌象】舌苔黄而干燥，满舌厚积，颗粒粗而疏松。望之如砂石，扪之糙手，望之苍老，舌质红绛。若苔黄而干涩，中有裂纹使之成为豆瓣状，称为“黄瓣苔”。

【主病】实热津伤。此舌属里热亢盛，热盛伤津之象。因热邪亢盛熏蒸于舌故苔呈黄色，热邪伤津，故苔干燥不润，甚则糙裂如砂石。

【治法】清热生津；苦寒攻下。

2. The Thick, Dry and Yellow Coating(Figure 6.9)

【Manifestations】The coating is yellow, dry and thickness fully distributed on the whole tongue. The grains of coating are loose, seeming as sands and feeling rough. The color of tongue proper is red crimson. Since the dry yellow coating has a split in the middle, which divides the tongue surface into two half, as if two pieces of one pea, the coating is called “yellow pea-like coating”.

【Indications】Consumption of the body fluid by excessive heat. This is a sign of impairment of the body fluid by excessive interior-heat, which is so exuberant that flaring upward to the tongue. As a result the coating is affected as yellow color. Since the body fluid has been consumed by pathogenic heat, it can not provide enough nourishment, bringing the tongue dryness and rough like sands.

【Treatment】To clear away heat and promote production of fluid, or to purge the bowels with bitter and cold herbs.

3. **焦黄苔**(图 6.10)

【舌象】苔色黄灰黑相兼，苔质干燥糙裂，如烧焦烤糊之锅巴，舌质红。

【主病】胃肠热结(阳明腑实证)。

这种舌象的形成与黄燥苔基本相同,只是程度更甚。中医学认为,邪热内盛,如果大小便通畅,则邪热可随二便而出,即邪热尚有出路。如若邪热太甚,胃肠津伤,热邪与肠中燥屎互结在一起致使大便秘结不通,就会将邪热闭郁于体内不得外出,这样就会造成里热越盛、津液越伤、津越伤大便越秘结不通的恶性循环,人体好像成了一个密闭的大烤炉,将一切都烤得焦干,舌苔即呈现出焦黄色。

【治法】苦寒直折,急下存阴。

3. The Black Yellow Coating(Figure 6.10)

【Manifestations】The color of coating is a gathering of yellow, gray and black. The property of fur is dry, rough and fissured as though scorched crispy rice, and tongue color is red.

【Indications】Accumulation of heat in the gastrointestinal tract. The formation of the tongue picture is similar to that of yellow dryness coating, only in a more serious stage. According to TCM, the excess heat in the interior can be expelled out of the body through defecation and urination. But if the heat in the interior is too heavy to dispel, it will stagnate in the interior and consume the body fluid, leading to constipation. In turn, obstruction of bowel movement will promote pathogenic heat more serious and make the disease worse. Under such a condition, the body is burned and scorched by the intense heat in the same way as an oven, and finally the color of coating is made into black yellow.

【Treatment】To clear away heat by purging swiftly with bitter and cold herbs, and promote production of fluid.

4. **黄腻苔(图** 6.11)

【舌象】苔色黄而粘腻不干,颗粒紧密胶粘,与舌质紧密相连,不易刮去。

【主病】湿热痰涎交结为患。苔黄为热,苔腻为湿、为痰、为食滞,故黄腻苔主湿热交结、痰热互结、食滞化热等证。如黄色深,粘腻程度较重的,是热重于湿,痰涎之邪亦甚;如黄色浅,粘腻程度较轻的,是湿重于热,痰涎之邪亦轻。

【治法】清热化湿祛痰。

4. The Yellow and Greasy Coating(Figure 6.11)

【Manifestations】The yellow and greasy coating sticks to the tongue proper tightly in difficulty to scrape off.

【Indications】The syndrome of dampness heat and phlegm. Usually the yellow coating means heat, while greasy means dampness phlegm or food retention. So the yellow and greasy coating reflects the combination of pathogenic dampness with heat, or phlegm with heat, or retention of food heat. If the coating is deep yellow and obviously sticky, it means that heat pathogen is severer than dampness. But if the coating is slight yellow and mild greasy, it suggests that dampness is heavier than heat.

【Treatment】To clear away heat as well as to eliminate dampness and phlegm.

5. 淡黄滑苔(图 6.12)

【舌象】舌苔淡黄,舌质淡白胖嫩,有裂纹。

【主病】脾肾阳虚,湿郁化热。

此舌象多由阳虚土败,寒湿、痰饮内停,若伴有阳虚血瘀还可见舌色淡白滞暗。

【治法】温阳化饮,兼以清热。

5. The Light Yellow and Watery Coating(Figure 6.12)

【Manifestations】The color of coating is yellowish. The tongue proper is pale, puffy, tender, and fissured.

【Indications】Deficiency of the spleen-kidney Yang, as well as dampness heat due to retention. Because of deficiency of the spleen and kidney Yang, cold dampness phlegm come into being and accumulate in the interior. Over a long period the retention will transform into heat. This heat belongs to deficient heat and it is not intense, so bringing the coating light yellow color. Owing to the cold dampness retention, the surface of tongue shows watery and even drips saliva. If the disease is complicated with blood stasis caused by Yang deficiency, the tongue may appear pale and dim.

【Treatment】To warm Yang and resolve phlegm as well as to clear away heat.

三、灰、黑苔

灰苔与黑苔同类，苔色呈浅黑时即为灰，苔色呈深灰时即为黑，因而灰黑苔可以相并而论。病至苔色灰黑，一般病都比较严重，均为里证，无表证。临证只凭灰黑苔色尚不能辨别其证属虚、实、寒、热，还必须结合舌质的形色和苔质的情况具体分析，其中苔质的润燥是鉴别灰黑苔寒热属性的重要指征。

一般认为黑苔主热极或寒盛之危证。若舌苔黑而水湿滑润，多属阳虚寒盛，湿邪伤脾，这种舌象的形成以淡白舌白滑苔为基础，是从这种舌象发展演变而来的。若舌苔灰黑而干燥糙裂，舌质红绛，甚则芒刺满布，多属热炽津伤，少阴真水将涸，火极似水（五行学说中肾属水，五色配黑）之候，这种舌象的形成是从红绛舌干黄苔发展而来，故为热极之征。

常见灰黑苔及主病如下。

Ⅲ. The Gray and Black Coating

The gray coating is similar to the black coating, but is slight in color. With the gray and black coating the illness is usually serious and belongs to the interior-syndrome. No exterior-syndrome presents the coating like that. In clinic this kind of coating should be combined with the shape and color of the tongue body as well as coating proper so as to identify the deficiency, excess, cold or heat of diseases. The important manifestation for judgment is whether moistness on the tongue, which can tell cold nature from heat during illness.

Generally, the black coating manifests critical syndrome of extreme heat or excessive cold. In detail, the black coating showing watery reflects excessive cold due to Yang deficiency, as well as injury of the spleen by the dampness. Usually the tongue as above is developed from the white moist coating with pale tongue. But when the gray-black coating is dry, rough and fissured and accompanied by the red crimson tongue proper or even with prickles, it reflects exhaustion of Yin fluid by extreme heat pathogen. This is developed from the dry, yellow coating and crimson tongue.

The common black and gray coatings and their indications in clinic are as follows.

1. **焦黑干燥苔**(图 6.13)

【舌象】苔质焦黑,干燥糙裂,舌质红,边光剥。

【主病】热极津伤。实热极盛,燔灼焚焰,故苔黑而干焦,舌质红绛。若苔黑而燥裂,舌质紫绛生芒刺,是热极津枯。

【治法】清热生津;苦寒攻下。

1. Dry and Black Coating(Figure 6.13)

【Manifestations】 The coating of tongue is scorched-like blackness and also rough dryness marked by fissures. The tongue proper is red, with no coating at all on sides of the tongue.

【Indications】 Depletion of the body fluid by extreme heat. The crimson tongue and black dryness coating result from flaring up of hyperactive fire. If the coating is black and rough with fissures, and the tongue proper is deep purple with thorns, it means exhaustion of the body fluid by extreme heat.

【Treatment】 To promote production of body fluid and clear away heat by purging bowels with bitter and cold herbs.

2. **白腻灰黑苔**(图 6.14)

【舌象】舌苔白腻,日久不化,从舌中、根部渐现灰黑苔,舌面湿润,舌边尖处仍为白腻苔,舌质淡白胖嫩。

【主病】阳虚寒湿。此舌象为虚寒夹湿,尤多见于脾阳不振,水饮内停的病变。

【治法】温中散寒。

2. The White Greasy and Gray Darkness Coating(Figure 6.14)

【Manifestations】 The coating keeps white greasy coating for long period, and gradually appears gray black color and moisture in the middle and root region. On the sides and tip there are still white and greasy coating left. The tongue proper is pale, puffy and tender.

【Indications】 This is a symptom of fluid retention due to deficient cold, usually seen in the case of spleen-Yang deficiency, which causes accumulation of water dampness.

【Treatment】 To warm the middle-Yang and dispel cold dampness.

应当指出,黑苔还可因 瘀血、吸烟等引起,故并不一定标志病情危重,所以临证时还要注意四诊合参,只要舌质红活荣润,运动灵活,无紫晦、干枯、无神等改变,均非病情危重。

At last, it should be pointed out that the black coating is possible to occur within blood-stagnation or smoking. In case of that, it is not the mark of critical condition. Therefore it should be paid more attention to comprehend the four diagnostic methods in clinic and make correct differentiation. In short, when the tongue body is light red, vitality, and moisture, moving freely, with no signs of dark purple, or dry rough, or flaccid appearance, it doesn't meat serious diseases.

第2部分　临床篇

PART TWO　CLINIC

第 7 章 淡白舌

1. 淡白红点舌,薄白苔(图 7.1)

【舌象】舌质淡白,舌边尖有红点,舌苔薄白。

【主病】素体虚弱,复感温热邪气,邪客于表。平素正气不足,气血虚弱,血液不能充分营运于舌质之中,而致舌质淡白不红。温热邪气初犯于表,尚未入里,对脏腑功能的影响未深,故舌苔薄白。温热邪气蕴于血分,有透表之势,则舌的边尖见红点。常见于身体虚弱,如患有慢性消化系统疾病,贫血等患者并发急性感染,或流行性感冒的初期。

【治疗】宜先以辛凉解表为主治疗,常用方药为银翘散。

【针刺取穴】合谷、列缺、曲池、大椎、风池、足三里。

Chapter 7 The Pale Tongue(Figure 7.1)

1. The Pale Tongue with Red Spots, Covered by Thin White Fur

【Manifestations】The tongue is pale, with some red spots on the sides and tip, covered by white and thin coating.

【Indications】 The weakened constitution is complicated with invasion of warm-heat pathogen to the exterior. The vital Qi of the body is usually insufficient, and Qi-blood is weak. The blood can not fully flow into the tongue body for its nourishment, leaving the tongue pale and less red in color. The warm-heat pathogen newly attacks the exterior of the body and hasn't transmitted into the interior. It gives no obvious disturbance to the viscera, therefore the tongue coating shows thin and white. Otherwise, warm-heat pathogen stagnates in the blood system, tending to penetrate outwards, bringing some red spots on the border and tip of tongue. It is often seen in the cases of weakness constitution suffering from chronic diseases of the digestive system, or anemia with acute infection, or initial stage of flu.

【Treatment】 Firstly, treatment should aim at relieving exterior syndrome with acrid and cool herbs. Yin-Qiao-San(银翘散) is commonly used.

【Selection of acupoints】Hegu(LI4), Lieque(Lu7), Quchi(LI11), Dazhui(Du14), Fengchi(GB20), Zusanli(St36).

2. 淡白舌,薄白腻苔(图 7.2)

【舌象】舌质淡白,舌苔薄白腻,根部略见黄色。

【主病】正气虚损,湿浊不化。薄苔主外感表证或内伤轻病。白腻不燥,为湿浊内停的表现,根部略见黄色,说明湿浊有化热的趋势。舌质淡白主虚、主寒。本舌象提示为内有虚寒,运化无力,湿浊不化之轻症。本舌象见于慢性胃炎、十二指肠溃疡、消化不良以及流行性感冒、神经衰弱等症,中医辨证为虚寒湿浊不化。

【治疗】健脾利湿。方用参苓白术散。

【针刺取穴】足三里、中脘、天枢、阴陵泉、三阴交、脾俞、三焦俞。

2. The Pale Tongue Covered with Thin, White and Sticky Fur(Figure 7.2)

【Manifestations】 The tongue is pale. The coating is thin, white and sticky, with light yellow color seen at the root.

【Indications】 It suggests the syndrome of vital Qi weakness and dampness retention. The thin coating indicates the exterior syndrome, or mild diseases of the internal injury. The white, sticky coating with no dryness is a manifestation of turbid dampness stagnating in the interior. Light yellow color seen at the root of the tongue implies that there is a tendency to heat transformed from turbid dampness. Usually, the pale tongue reflects the syndromes of deficiency and cold, so the tongue manifestation as above suggests a mild case of dampness retention due to internal deficient cold that leads to a weakened transformation and transportation. It is commonly seen in the cases of chronic gastritis, duodenum ulcer, dyspepsia, and flu, or neurasthenia, etc., which are differentiated by traditional Chinese medicine as the syndrome of dampness retention due to deficient cold.

【Treatment】 The method is to invigorate the spleen and resolve dampness. Shen-Ling-Bai-Zhu-San(参苓白术散) can be used.

【Selection of acupoints】Zusanli (St36), Zhongwan (Ren12), Tianshu (St25), Yinlingquan (Sp9), Sanyinjiao (Sp6), Pishu(UB20), Sanjiaoshu(UB22).

3. 淡白舌,白滑苔(图7.3)

【舌象】舌质淡白,舌苔白腻而略滑。

【主病】阳气不足,寒湿内停。阳气不足,无力鼓动血行。气血不能充分营运于舌中,致舌质淡白不红。阳虚里寒,气化失司,水液代谢障碍,水湿痰浊停于体内,反映于舌,则见舌苔白腻略滑,痰稀白。常见于慢性支气管炎、慢性肾小球肾炎、肾病综合征等病症。

【治疗】以温振阳气,运化水湿为主。以脾阳不足,大便泄泻为主者,方用附子理中汤。

【针刺取穴】天枢、气海、足三里、阴陵泉、太溪、脾俞、肾俞。

3. The Pale Tongue with white and watery coating(Figure 7.3)

【Manifestations】 The tongue is pale. The coating is white, sticky and slightly watery.

【Indications】 It reflects that Yang Qi is insufficient and cold dampness accumulates in the interior. Since deficient Yang Qi is weak in promoting blood circulation normally, Qi and blood can not fully flow up to the tongue and give enough nourishment, leading to the pale tongue with less red. On the other hand, deficient Yang Qi causes the interior cold, which makes the disorder of water metabolism, bringing about retention of water dampness and phlegm that can be reflected by the white, sticky and slightly watery coating. The sputum is thin and white. This kind of the tongue is often seen in diseases of chronic bronchitis, chronic glomerulonephritis, nephrotic syndrome, and so on.

【Treatment】 The main treatment principle is to warm Yang and resolve dampness. In case of the spleen Yang deficiency marked by diarrhoea, Fu-Zi-Li-Zhong-Tang(附子理中汤) should be adopted.

【Selection of acupoints】Tianshu (St25), Qihai (Ren6), Zusanli (St36), Yinlingquan (Sp9), Taixi (K3), Pishu (UB20), Shenshu (UB23).

4. 淡白黑点舌,薄白根腻苔(图 7.4)

【舌象】舌质淡白偏暗滞,舌体胖嫩,边尖有黑点;舌苔薄白而腻,根部略显淡黄。

【主病】脾阳不振,心血瘀阻。脾阳不足,故气血不能充分营运于舌,以致舌色淡白暗滞;舌体胖大,舌苔白腻是脾虚不能运化水湿之故;湿蕴血瘀,有化热之势,故舌见黑点和淡黄苔。可见于心脏病、胃及十二指肠溃疡等消化系统疾病患者,症见心悸虚烦,面色无华,纳呆口干,神疲乏力,身重肢肿。

【治疗】法当温阳益气,活血利水。方用真武汤加减。

【针刺取穴】合谷、太冲、气海、天枢、阴陵泉、足三里、中脘、内关、太溪。

4. The Pale Tongue with Black Spots, Covered by Thin White Fur as well as Sticky Fur Seen at the Root(Figure 7.4)

【Manifestations】 The tongue is pale, slightly dim and dull. The body of the tongue is enlarged and tender with some black spots on the sides and tip. The coating is thin white and sticky, at the root, showing light yellow color.

【Indications】 It indicates deficient spleen Yang and heart blood stasis. The spleen Yang is insufficient and failure in promoting blood circulation fully up to the tongue for enough nourishment, so bringing the tongue into pale, dark and dull appearance. The enlarged tongue body and white sticky coating are caused by water dampness retention due to poor function of deficient spleen Yang in transformation and transportation. On the other hand, dampness retention can cause blood stasis. The stagnancy can transform into heat, giving rise to some black spots on the tongue as well as light yellow coating. It may occur in cases of heart diseases or digestive system diseases, such as gastroduodenal ulcer, marked by palpitation, restlessness, pale complexion, poor appetite, and dryness in the mouth, lassitude, swollen limbs, as well as heavy sensation of body.

【Treatment】The method should be warming Yang and reinforcing Qi, combined with promoting blood circulation and excreting water dampness. Modified Zhen-Wu-Tang(真武汤)can be used.

【Selection of acupoints】Hegu(LI4), Taichong(Liv3), Qihai(Ren6), Tianshu(St25), Yinlingquan(Sp9), Zusanli(St36), Zhongwan(Ren12), Neiguan(P6), Taixi(K3).

5. 淡白舌,白厚苔(图 7.5)

【舌象】舌质淡白,舌苔白厚。

【主病】正气虚弱,湿邪内盛,或表邪入里。舌质淡白提示正气不足,身体虚弱。舌苔的厚薄变化,主要反映邪正的盛衰。厚苔是胃气挟湿浊邪气熏蒸而成,在内伤病中见厚苔,主内有痰湿或食积;在外感病中见厚苔,主邪气盛,已由表入里,为病进。苔质虽厚而色白,表明邪气虽盛,但尚未化热。

【治疗】脾胃虚弱,复有食积或湿浊内停者,可选用香砂六君子汤。

【针刺取穴】中脘、天枢、肓俞、足三里、丰隆、阳陵泉、太冲。

5. The pale Tongue with White and Thick Fur(Figure 7.5)

【Manifestations】The tongue is pale, and the coating is white and thick.

【Indications】It indicates either deficient vital Qi with excess internal dampness or invasion of exogenous pathogens to the interior. The pale tongue suggests that vital Qi is insufficient, and constitution is weak. Changes of the thickness on the coating can reflect conditions of both pathogen and vital Qi. The thick coating is formed by a steaming action of the stomach Qi in combination with turbid dampness. So it means dampness phlegm or indigested food retention in the interior seen in case of the internal injury. But occurring in the exogenous disease, it means pathogens excessively invading the interior from the exterior, and diseases aggravating. The coating is thick but still white, suggesting no heat transformed from the excessive pathogens yet.

【Treatment】For the deficient spleen-stomach complicated with food retention or turbid dampness, Xiang-Sha-Liu-Jun-Zi-Tang(香砂六君子汤)can be chosen.

【Selection of acupoints】Zhongwan (Ren12), Tianshu (St25), Huangshu (K16), Zusanli (St36), Fenglong (St40), Yanglingquan(GB34), Taichong(Liv3).

6. 淡白略暗舌,薄白淡黄苔(图 7.6)

【舌象】舌质淡白偏暗(略带青紫色),苔薄色黄中部较明显。

【主病】正虚夹热,轻度瘀滞。正气虚弱,气血不足见舌质淡白。气虚运行无力,血脉又见轻度瘀滞,故舌带青紫色而略偏暗。里有热邪但不甚,故苔薄黄;微热居中焦脾胃,故舌中部明显。本舌象提示正虚感受热邪,或伤寒初入阳明,或正虚伴有食滞,中焦脾胃郁热上蒸。本舌象常可见于现代医学的传染性及感染性发热的疾病,如流行性感冒、上呼吸道感染、胃肠炎、神经官能症、高血压等疾病。

【治疗】清胃热,理气血。药用清胃散。

【针刺取穴】合谷、太冲、足三里、关元、中脘、曲池、阳陵泉。

6. The Pale and Dim Tongue Covered by the Thin White and Light Yellow Coating(Figure 7.6)

【Manifestations】The tongue is pale, dark and bluish purple, covered by thin coating with an obvious yellow color in its center.

【Indications】It denotes deficiency of vital Qi with heat pathogen in combination of mild blood stasis. Weakness of vital Qi and Qi-blood deficiency may show the tongue pale. Weakened Qi is not sufficient enough to promote blood circulation normally, leading to mild stasis of blood. So the tongue shows bluish purple and darkness. Heat pathogen exists in the interior but it is not intense, therefore bringing a thin yellow coating. The heat pathogen is located in the middle-jiao producing an obvious yellow in the center of the tongue. This tongue picture indicates vital Qi deficiency attacked by exogenous heat pathogen, or febrile disease newly affecting Yang-Ming, or deficiency of vital Qi complicated with food stagnation that causes stagnant heat steaming upwards from the spleen and stomach of the middle-Jiao. The picture as above is often seen in terms of modern medicine of epidemic disease, and infectious febrile diseases, such as flu, upper respiratory tract infection, gastroenteritis, neurosis, hypertension, etc.

【Treatment】 To clear away the stomach heat and regulate Qi and blood. Qing-Wei-San(清胃散) can be used.

【Selection of acupoints】Hegu(LI4), Taichong(Liv3), Zusanli(St36), Guanyuan(Ren4), Zhongwan(Ren12), Quchi (LI11), Yanglingquan(GB34).

7. 淡白偏暗舌,薄白根黄苔(图7.7)

【舌象】舌质淡白偏暗,舌苔薄白根部略黄腻。

【主病】阳虚气虚又感外邪。患者素体阳气虚弱,不能温运气血,表现于舌色上可见舌质淡白而暗滞,苔白也主寒证,根部已现淡黄腻,说明邪气有化热的倾向。可见于气虚感冒初起的患者。

【治疗】益气解表,调和营卫。方用参苏饮加味。

【针刺取穴】中脘、天枢、合谷、列缺、曲池、足三里、关元。

7. The Pale Dark Tongue Covered by Thin White Fur with Yellow Color at the Root(Figure 7.7)

【Manifestations】 The tongue is pale and dark. The coating is thin and white and shows mild yellow sticky at the root.

【Indications】 It is regarded as deficiency of both Yang and Qi attacked by exogenous pathogen. The patient is usually weak in Yang-Qi and warming and leading blood circulation, which is manifested as the pale tongue with darkness and dull appearance. The white coating is also attributable to cold syndrome. At the root of tongue, light yellow and sticky coating occurring means a tendency to heat transformed from pathogen. The tongue is usually seen in the case of the early stage of common cold due to Qi deficiency.

【Treatment】 To reinforce Qi and relieve the exterior, as well as to harmonize Ying and Wei(nutrient Qi and defensive Qi). The prescription should apply modified Shen-Su-Yin(参苏饮).

【Selection of acupoints】 Zhongwan (Ren12), Tianshu (St25), Quchi(LⅢ), Hegu(LI4), Lieque(Lu7), Quchi(LI11), Zusanli (St36), Guanyuan(Ren4).

8. 淡白裂纹舌,偏黄浮垢苔(图 7.8)

【舌象】舌质淡白有裂纹,舌根部有偏黄浮垢苔,舌面干。

【主病】气阴两虚,湿浊不化。多见于久病脏腑功能减退,阴液大伤,仍有湿热之邪内停。舌质淡白略胖为素体阳气亏虚,舌体有裂纹为阴液亏损,舌根部有偏黄浮垢苔为湿热之邪未化之证。大便干燥,小便短少,脉细无力。临床常见慢性气管炎、肺心病或膀胱炎、盆腔炎等慢性疾病的急性发作,也可见于急性传染病,如乙脑、肠伤寒等病的恢复期,以及癌症、血液病、结缔组织病,内分泌系统疾病所引起的发热、植物神经功能紊乱所致的低热,而中医辨证为气阴两虚,湿浊不化。

【治疗】补益气血,药用归脾汤。

【针刺取穴】阳陵泉、三阴交、太溪、足三里、气海、天枢、曲池、太冲。

8. The Pale and Fissured Tongue with a Layer of Yellow, Floating and Turbid Fur(Figure 7.8)

【Manifestations】 The tongue is pale and fissured. There is light yellow, floating and turbid coating at the root. On the surface, it shows dryness.

【Indications】 It indicates a syndrome of deficient Qi and Yin as well as dampness retention. This is usually seen in some prolonged diseases with dysfunction of viscera and exhaustion of

Yin fluid in combination with internal dampness heat. The pale and puffy tongue means an usual deficiency of Yang and Qi. Fissures of the tongue mark exhaustion of Yin fluid. And the light yellow, floating and turbid coating at the root is a sign of dampness heat which is not resolved. The symptoms linked with the tongue may be dry stools, scanty urine, thready and weak pulse. The syndrome is often seen on acute attack of some chronic diseases, such as tracheitis, pulmonary heart disease, or cystitis, and pelvic inflammation. It is also seen in some acute diseases, such as restoring stage of encephalitis B or ileotyphus, as well as fever caused by cancer, hematopathy, connective tissue disease, and endocrine system disease, or low fever due to dysfunction of vegetative nerve. All of those are differentiated as deficiency of both Qi and Yin with retention of dampness turbidity by traditional Chinese medicine.

【Treatment】To reinforce Qi and replenish blood. Gui-Pi-Tang(归脾汤)can be used.

【Selection of acupoints】Yanglingquan(GB34), Sanyinjiao(Sp6), Taixi(K3), Zusanli(St36), Qihai(Ren6), Tianshu(St25), Quchi(LI11), Taichong(Liv3).

9. 淡白偏暗舌,根部浮垢苔(图7.9)

【舌象】舌质淡白有短小的鹅卵石状的裂纹,舌苔薄而透明,根部浮垢。

【主病】气血亏虚,又挟湿浊。舌面出现多少不等,各种形态明显的裂沟,总属阴血亏损,不能荣润舌面所致。根部苔质浮垢,说明内有湿浊之气为患,部位偏于下焦;若原来患者腐垢苔遍布舌面,或由板滞不宣而化腐,渐而退减到舌根部,这是正气胜邪的苔象。

本舌象可见于现代医学的高血压、贫血兼消化不良、慢性肾盂肾炎、慢性心功能不全的患者。

【治疗】补益气血,温阳利湿。药用当归补血汤和真武汤加减。

【针刺取穴】足三里、阳陵泉、阴陵泉、三阴交、太溪、气海、肾俞、脾俞。

9. The Pale and Dim Tongue with Floating Turbid Fur at

the Root(Figure 7.9)

【Manifestations】 The tongue is pale with some fissures in a cobble shape. The coating is thin and transparent, at its root part, you can see loose turbidity.

【Indications】 This picture suggests deficient Qi and blood as well as turbid dampness. The tongue shows some obvious fissures as a result of insufficient Yin blood in nourishing the tongue. At the root, there is loose turbidity coating, meaning dampness turbidity in the lower-Jiao. If the coating changes from the full surface of tongue to the root, or from tough and sticky to curdy appearance, it suggests the restored vital Qi overcoming pathogens. The picture as above can be seen in terms of modern medicine as hypertension, anemia with dyspepsia, chronic pyelonephritis, and chronic heart failure, etc.

【Treatment】 To benefit Qi and blood as well as to warm Yang and excrete dampness. Modified Dang-Gui-Bu-Xue-Tang (当归补血汤) with Zhen-Wu-Tang(真武汤) can be chosen.

【Selection of acupoints】 Zusanli (St36), Yanglingquan (GB34), Yinlingquan(Sp9), Sanyinjiao(Sp6), Taixi(K3), Qihai (Ren6), Pishu(UB20), Shenshu(UB23).

10. 淡白红点舌,白腻中黄苔(图 7.10)

【舌象】舌质淡白,边尖有红点,舌苔白腻,舌中部苔色微黄。

【主病】正气不足,脾胃虚弱,外感湿热邪气,邪气郁阻于中焦。平素中焦脾胃虚弱,气血化生无源,故见舌质淡白。感受湿热邪气,湿阻气机,气化不利,湿浊内停反映于舌则见腻苔。湿浊化热,则舌见红点,苔色淡黄。不欲饮,胸脘痞闷等症。可见于虚人外感湿温或暑湿困脾等。

【治疗】治以化湿清热,可用三仁汤。

【针刺取穴】中脘、天枢、足三里、阳陵泉、丰隆、曲池、合谷、气海。

10. The Pale Tongue with Red Spots, Covered by White and Sticky Fur, Showing Yellow Fur in the Middle Part(Figure 7.10)

【Manifestations】The tongue is pale, some red spots seen on its sides and tip. The coating is white and sticky in light yellow color in the center.

【Indications】It is produced by deficiency of vital Qi and the spleen-stomach, complicated with exogenous dampness heat that stagnates in the middle-Jiao. Usually the spleen and stomach of the middle-Jiao are insufficient, Qi and blood generated is insufficient, giving rise to the tongue pale in color. Because of attack by pathogenic dampness heat that obstructs functional activity of Qi, the Qi transformation is disordered, leading to retention of internal damp turbidity, reflected by the sticky coating. Turbid dampness transforms into heat and brings red spots of the tongue and light yellow coating. The symptoms may be no desire for drinking, stuffiness and distention over the chest and stomach. It can occur in the debility case invaded by exogenous warm dampness, or summer heat dampness obstructing the spleen, etc.

【Treatment】The method is to resolve dampness and clear away heat. San-Ren-Tang(三仁汤) can be used.

【Selection of acupoints】Zhongwan (Ren12), Tianshu (St25), Zusanli (St36), Yanglingquan (GB34), Fenglong (St40), Quchi(LI11), Hegu(LI4), Qihai(Ren6).

11. 淡白瘀斑舌,双黄苔(图7.11)

【舌象】舌质淡白偏暗,舌边有瘀斑,舌苔薄白,内夹两条黄苔。

【主病】气虚血瘀,脾胃湿热。瘀斑是血脉瘀滞之象。舌上两条黄苔,说明体内邪热上攻,是脾胃湿热的表现。本舌象提示患者因气虚,使脾胃转输不利,推动血脉运行不利,所以不仅见到舌质淡白的本虚之象,同时伴有血瘀、湿热内蕴的标象。口干,大便小爽,脉迟。本古象常见于现代医字的慢性胃炎,十二指肠溃疡,神经衰弱,心功能不全,高血压等病症,中医辨证为气虚血瘀,脾胃湿热。

【治疗】补气养血活血,清热健脾祛湿。药用参苓白术散。

【针刺取穴】合谷、太冲、三阴交、中脘、天枢、气海、足三里。

11. The Pale and Petechia Tongue Covered by White Fur with Double Yellow Fur(Figure 7.11)

【Manifestations】 The tongue is pale and dim, showing purple marks on the border. The coating is thin and white with two pieces of yellow coatings on the surface.

【Indications】 It is formed by Qi deficiency and blood stasis in combination with dampness heat in the spleen and stomach. Purple spots are the sign of blockage of blood vessels. The coating with a pair of yellow pieces indicates pathogenic heat attacking upward, which is a manifestation of dampness heat in the spleen and stomach. This tongue picture denotes that because of Qi deficiency, the spleen and stomach are dysfunction in transportation, and blood circulates abnormally. So the tongue shows deficiency sign as well as stagnant appearance of both blood and dampness heat. The symptoms may be dryness in the mouth, dysuria, and slow pulse. This kind of tongue can be seen in chronic gastritis, duodenum ulcer, neurasthenia, heart failure, hypertension, and so on, which are differentiated by traditional Chinese medicine as Qi deficiency and blood stasis complicated with dampness heat in the spleen and stomach.

【Treatment】 The method should be strengthening Qi and nourishing blood, promoting blood circulation, as well as invigorating the spleen to expel dampness and clear away heat. The prescription should be modified Sen-Ling-Bai-Zhu-San(参苓白术散).

【Selection of acupoints】 Hegu(LI4), Taichong(Liv3), Sanyinjiao(Sp6), Zhongwan(Ren12), Tianshu(St25), Qihai (Ren6), Zusanli(St36).

12. **淡白齿痕舌,薄白双黄苔(图** 7.12)

【舌象】舌质淡白,边有齿痕,苔薄白,舌两侧均有条状淡黄苔,称为双黄苔。

【主病】脾虚湿盛,湿郁化热。常见于素体脾虚不能运化水湿。湿邪久留化热,湿热蕴结于脾胃、肝胆。舌边有齿痕为脾气虚弱，水湿内聚。双黄苔为湿热蕴结肝胆、脾胃，临床可见急性发热性疾患，如感冒、流感之初、中期或胆结石、慢性胆囊炎急性发作。

【治疗】利湿清热。①湿热蕴积肝胆者，清利肝胆湿热之法，药用黄芩滑石汤加减。②热在肺胃，可用新加白虎汤加减，以辛凉泄热。③如邪在半表半里，出入于表里之间，可用和解少阳的方法，用小柴胡汤加减或用成药舒肝和胃丸、藿香正气丸。

【针刺取穴】曲池、合谷、阳陵泉、足三里、太冲、三阴交、阴陵泉、肝俞、胆俞。

12. The Pale Tongue with Tooth Traces, Covered by Thin and White Fur, Showing Double Yellow Coatings on the Bilateral Sides(Figure 7.12)

【Manifestations】 The tongue is pale with tooth marks at its edges, covered by thin and white coating as well as yellow coating on both sides, which is termed double yellow coating.

【Indications】 It indicates the spleen deficiency and dampness excess that accumulates and transforms into heat. It is usually seen in the case of the spleen insufficiency and failure in transporting water dampness. When dampness accumulates for a long time, it can transform into heat. Dampness heat may stagnate in the spleen and stomach, or in the liver and gallbladder. The tongue has tooth traces, it means deficiency of the spleen Qi as well as retention of water dampness in the interior. The double yellow coating reflects dampness heat stagnating in the liver-gallbladder, or in the spleen-stomach. Clinically, it is seen in acute febrile diseases, such as the early or middle stage of flu, or gallstone, or acute attack of chronic cholecystitis.

【Treatment】 To excrete dampness and clear away heat. (1) For the syndrome of dampness heat stagnating in the liver and gallbladder, treatment should be to eliminate damp heat from the liver and gallbladder. Modified Huang-Qin-Hua-Shi-Tang(黄芩滑石汤) can be applied. (2) For the syndrome of heat in the lung and stomach, modified Xin-Jia-Bai-Hu-Tang (新加白虎汤) can be chosen to eliminate heat with acrid and cool herbs. (3) For the syndrome of pathogen between the exterior and interior, harmonizing therapy should be applied and modified Xiao-Chai-Hu-Tang(小柴胡汤) can be used. Proprietary medicines, such as Shu-Gan-Hu-Wei-Wan(舒肝和胃丸) or Huo-Xiang-Zheng-Qi-Wan(藿香正气丸) can be used.

【Selection of acupoints】 Quchi(LI11), Hegu(LI4), Zusanli(St36), Taichong(Liv3), Sanyinjiao(Sp6), Yinlingquan(Sp9), Ganshu(UB18), Danshu(UB19).

13. 淡白偏暗舌,白腻双黄苔(图 7.13)

【舌象】舌质淡白偏暗,舌尖有红色星点,苔薄白腻,内夹两条黄苔。

【主病】脾胃气虚,湿浊不化,郁而生热。脾虚运化不利,胃之浊气,久蕴化热,邪热上蒸,舌苔白腻,内夹两条黄苔,舌尖红点,说明湿滞化热,热在心脾。本舌象见于现代医学的慢性胃炎、胃神经官能症、消化不良、贫血等疾病患者。

【治疗】健胃益脾,化浊清热。药用六和汤。

【针刺取穴】中脘、太冲、气海、足三里、阳陵泉、曲池、合谷。

13. The Pale and Dim Tongue Covered by White and Sticky Fur with Double Yellow Furs(Figure 7.13)

【Manifestations】 The tongue is pale and dark, some red dots can been seen on its tip. The coating is thin, white and sticky with two yellow coatings.

【Indications】 It is caused by deficiency of the spleen-stomach Qi, accumulation of damp turbidity, and heat transformed from dampness stagnancy. The spleen is deficiency and failure in transformation and transportation, leaving the turbid Qi stagnated in the stomach and turned into heat after certain period. Pathogenic heat steams upwards, giving rise to the sticky whiteness coating with two pieces of yellow coatings. Red spots on the tip of tongue reflect pathogenic heat of the spleen and stomach transformed from damp turbidity. This kind of picture can be seen in terms of modern medicine as chronic gastritis, stomach neurosis, dyspepsia, and anemia, etc.

【Treatment】 The treatment therapy is to invigorate the spleen and benefit the stomach, in combination with resolving dampness and clearing away heat. Modified Liu-He-Tang(六和汤) can be chosen.

【Selection of acupoints】 Zhongwan (Ren12), Taichong (Liv3), Qihai (Ren6), Zusanli (St36), Yanglingquan (GB34), Quchi (LI11), Hegu (LI4).

14. 淡白偏暗舌,白腻根黄苔(图7.14)

【舌象】舌质淡白偏暗,舌体胖大,边有齿痕;舌苔白腻根部略见黄色。

【主病】阳气虚运化不利。舌色浅淡,色偏暗,说明阳气虚,推动血液运行能力减弱,血液运行受阻,血液不能畅达于舌,故有轻度瘀滞;阳气亏虚温化失权,体内水湿停留,久又可化热上扰,所以舌苔表现为白腻,根部见有黄色,说明病位在中下焦。由此舌象提示为阳气亏虚运化不利,有血瘀湿停的征象。本舌象常见于现代医学的轻度心功能不全和消化系统的炎性疾病,如慢性胃肠炎、慢性结肠炎、十二指肠溃疡、萎缩性胃炎,以及一些轻度感染性疾病,如贫血患者外感邪气入里或伤食化热。

【治疗】补气行血、清热利湿。方用六君子场合二妙丸。

【针刺取穴】脾俞、胃俞、肾俞、足三里、阴陵泉、三阴交、太溪、复溜。

14. The White Pale and a Bit Dark Tongue Covered by Sticky and White, Yellow Fur at the Root(Figure 7.14)

【Manifestations】 The tongue is pale and dim. Its body is enlarged with some tooth traces. The coating is sticky and white, at the root, it is light yellow.

【Indications】 It is attributed to Yang deficiency and dysfunction in transformation and transportation. The pale and dark color of the tongue suggests mild blood stagnation due to Yang deficiency that is weak in promoting blood circulation. Deficient Yang is failure in warming and distributing water dampness, which accumulates in the interior and further transforms into heat. Heat disturbs upwards, manifesting as sticky and white coating as well as yellow coating at the root that indicates the location of illness being the middle and lower-Jiao. Therefore the tongue picture shows the sign of dysfunction in transforming and transporting due to Yang deficiency as well as stagnancy of both blood and dampness. This kind of tongue is usually seen in terms of modern medicine, such as mild heart failure, chronic gastroenteritis, chronic colonitis, duodenum ulcer, atrophic gastritis, or some mild infectious disease, such as anemia suffering from the exterior syndrome, or suffering from food retention transforming into heat.

【Treatment】 The method should be strengthening Qi and promoting blood circulation, in combination with clearing away heat and excreting dampness. The prescription should be Liu-Jun-Zi-Tang(六君子汤) combined with Er-Miao-Wan(二妙丸).

【Selection of acupoints】 Pishu(UB20), Weishu(UB21), Shenshu(UB23), Zusanli(St36), Yinlingquan(Sp9), Sanyinjiao(Sp6), Taixi(K3), Fuliu(K7).

15. 淡白舌,白腻根黄苔(图 7.15)

【舌象】舌质淡白,舌苔白腻,根部苔黄。

【主病】阳虚里寒,湿浊内停。舌质淡白与白腻苔同时出现,提示机体内阳气不足,导致气化不利,水液代谢失调,寒湿、痰浊停于体内。根部苔黄,为湿浊久停,有化热的征兆。小便短少。常见于慢性肾小球肾炎、肾病综合征,心功能不全,内分泌失调,如甲状腺机能减退以及慢性营养不良等疾病。

【治疗】温补脾肾,利湿化浊,方用温脾汤。浮肿重在下部,腰酸腿软者,可选用济生肾气丸加减。

【针刺取穴】足三里、三阴交、阴陵泉、太溪、照海、中极、关元。

15. The Pale Tongue Covered by White and Sticky Fur with Yellow Appearance at the Root(Figure 7.15)

【Manifestations】 The tongue is pale. The fur is white and sticky, yellow coating exists at the root.

【Indications】 It is produced by internal cold due to Yang

deficiency and dampness retention. When the pale tongue is present together with white and sticky coating, it suggests that Yang is insufficient and dysfunction in Qi transformation as well as water metabolism, resulting in cold dampness and phlegm turbidity accumulated inside the body. The yellow coating seen at the root of the tongue is a sign of heat transformed from prolonged stagnation of dampness turbidity. This tongue picture is usually associated with scanty urine, and often occurs in diseases, such as chronic glomerulonephritis, nephrotic syndrome, cardiac insufficiency, disorder of endocrine, hypothyroidism, and chronic malnutrition, etc.

【Treatment】 The therapy is to warm and reinforce the spleen and kidney as well as excrete dampness and resolve turbidity. Modified Wen-Pi-Tang(温脾汤) should be chosen, or Ji-Sheng-Shen-Qi-Wan(济生肾气丸) can be used if somebody has edema in the lower part of the body, soreness of loins and weakness of legs.

【Selection of acupoints】 Zusanli(St36), Sanyinjiao(Sp6), Yinlingquan(Sp9), Taixi(K3), Zhaohai(K6), Zhongji(Ren3), Guanyuan(Ren4).

16. 淡白舌,白黄腻苔(图7.16)

【舌象】舌质淡白,舌苔腻,苔色黄白相兼。

【主病】正气不足,湿郁化热。舌质淡白见于气血虚弱或阳气不足之证,因正气不足,鼓动气血无力,故见舌质淡白少红。脏腑功能减退,则湿浊、痰饮、食积易于停滞于体内。湿浊内蕴,阳气进一步被遏,则可在淡白舌的基础上出现腻苔。苔色由白渐转黄,标志着湿浊邪气有郁而化热之势。发热而欲盖衣被,口渴喜热饮,常见于慢性肝炎迁延期、慢性支气管炎或哮喘的急性发作期,亦可见于虚证发热,如白血病时的发热等。

【治疗】原则以先祛邪,即化湿浊,泄郁热为主。

【针刺取穴】阳陵泉、足三里、阴陵泉、合谷、曲池。

16. The Pale Tongue with White, Yellow and Sticky Fur (Figure 7.16)

【Manifestations】 The tongue is pale. The coating is sticky, white and light yellow.

【Indications】 It results from deficient vital Qi and pathogenic heat from stagnant dampness. The pale tongue is frequently seen in the syndrome of Qi and blood deficiency as well as Yang Qi insufficient. Because vital Qi is insufficient, it fails to promote Qi and blood circulation normally, leading to the pale tongue with less red. The functions of viscera are weakened, so dampness turbidity, phlegm, and indigested food are easy to stagnate in the interior, which further obstruct Yang Qi, consequently bringing sticky coating on the base of pale tongue. The color of coating grows from white to yellow, indicating the heat tendency transformed from stagnant turbid dampness pathogen. The symptoms associated with the tongue may be fever but the patient desires more clothes and quilt, and feels thirst with preference for hot drinks. The tongue picture often occurs in persistent hepatitis, chronic bronchitis, or in acute onset of asthma, as well as in deficiency-heat, such as fever due to leukaemia, and so on.

【Treatment】 The principle is to expel pathogens firstly, i.e. mainly to resolve dampness turbidity and purge stagnant heat.

【Selection of acupoints】 Yanglingquan (GB34), Zusanli (St36), Yinlingquan (Sp9), Hegu (LI4), Quchi (LI11).

17. 淡白舌,黄腻苔(图 7.17)

【舌象】舌质淡白,舌苔腻中部色黄。

【主病】气血不足,湿热中阻。气为血帅,气虚则运血无力,可致舌色淡白。腻苔主湿浊、痰饮、食积、顽痰等,色黄是有热。舌苔中部黄腻,说明中焦脾胃有湿浊或食滞内停,郁而化热之象。由此提示本舌象为正气虚,又挟食滞或湿热浊气内蕴之症。脉细滑。食滞重者亦可见口臭,大便不爽。本舌象常可见于现代医学的消化系统疾病,如慢性胃肠炎、慢性结肠炎、消化不良。

【治疗】补益气血,清化湿浊,兼以行气。药用八珍汤合小陷胸汤加减运用。

【针刺取穴】中脘、天枢、气海、足三里、丰隆、阳陵泉。

17. The Pale Tongue with Yellow and Sticky Fur (Figure 7.17)

【Manifestations】The tongue is pale. The sticky coating shows yellow color in the center.

【Indications】It is seen in the case of deficient Qi and blood, complicated with dampness heat stagnating in the middle-Jiao. In TCM opinion, Qi is the commander of blood. If Qi is insufficient in promoting blood circulation, it will lead to the tongue pale in color. The sticky coating indicates dampness turbidity, phlegm fluid, indigested food, or stubborn phlegm, etc. The yellow color means heat, so the tongue shows yellow and sticky coating in the center, it reflects the heat tendency transformed from dampness turbidity or indigested food stagnated within the spleen-stomach of the middle-Jiao. Therefore, the tongue picture denotes that this is the syndrome of vital Qi deficiency, complicated with stagnancy of food or dampness heat turbidity in the interior. The pulse may be thready and slippery. In the severe case of food retention, foul breath, and unsmooth stools may be found. This type of picture is often seen in terms of modern medicine as some diseases in digestive system, such as chronic gastroenteritis, chronic colonitis, or dyspepsia, etc.

【Treatment】The method should be to benefit both Qi and blood, as well as to eliminate dampness turbidity, in combination with promoting flow of Qi. Modified Ba-Zhen-Tang (八珍汤) and Xiao-Xian-Xiong-Tang (小陷胸汤) can be used together for this syndrome.

【Selection of acupoints】Zhongwan (Ren12), Tianshu (St25), Qihai (Ren6), Zusanli (St36), Fenglong (St40), Yanglingquan (GB34).

18. **淡白舌,白腻中灰苔(图 7.18)**

【舌象】舌质淡白,舌苔白腻,舌中呈灰苔。

【主病】阳气不足,阴寒内盛,水饮痰浊内停。舌质淡白表明正气虚,舌苔灰白而腻标志着寒湿内盛,是一种本虚标实的舌象。常见于慢性病的急性发作期或加重期。舌中出现湿润的灰苔,其阳虚里寒的程度较单独出现白腻苔更加严重。喘促,咳痰稀白。常见于慢性肾小球肾炎、肾病综合征、慢性支气管炎、哮喘、慢性心功能不全、慢性肝炎等病症。

【治疗】以温补脾肾,利湿行水为主。可用真武汤加减治疗。待白灰腻苔逐渐化退,转为白苔时,可服用济生肾气丸或参苓白术散,以补肾健脾,培固正气。

【针刺取穴】三阴交、阴陵泉、足三里、太溪、复溜、气海、关元。

18. The Pale Tongue Covered by Sticky and White Fur with Gray Fur in the Middle(Figure 7.18)

【Manifestations】 The tongue is pale. The coating is sticky and white, gray color can been seen in the middle.

【Indications】 It indicates Yang deficiency, internal Yin cold excess and water dampness turbidity accumulated in the interior. The pale tongue means vital Qi deficiency, while the gray, white and sticky coating suggests cold dampness excess in the interior. This is the picture of deficiency at the "root" and excess in the "branch". It is usually seen in chronic diseases' stage of acute attack or exacerbation stage. If the moist and gray coating occurs in the tongue, it demotes the internal cold due to Yang deficiency more severe than that with the white and sticky coating. Asthma, cough and thin white sputum may appear. It often occurs in chronic glomerulonephritis, nephrotic syndrome, chronic bronchitis, asthma, chronic cardiac insufficiency, chronic hepatitis, etc.

【Treatment】 The method should be warming and invigorating the spleen and kidney, as well as excreting water dampness. Modified Zhen-Wu-Tang(真武汤)can be used. While the coating changes from gray and sticky to white, Ji-Shen-Shen-Qi-Wan(济生肾气丸), or Shen-Ling-Bai-Zhu-San(参苓白术散) may be adopted to reinforce the kidney and spleen and consolidate vital Qi.

【Selection of acupoints】Sanyinjiao(sP6), Yinlingquan(Sp9),Zusanli(St36),Taixi(K3), Fuliu(K7),Qihai(Ren6),

Guanyuan(Ren4).

19. 淡白暗滞舌,根部黄灰苔(图7.19)

【舌象】舌质淡白暗滞,尖边有少数红色星点,根部舌苔黄腻而灰黑。

【主病】脾肾两虚,内有积滞。苔黄为热,苔腻为湿、为痰、为食滞,黄腻苔常与痰湿热郁、食滞化热相关。脾肾两虚,可使水液代谢障碍,积滞于内,下焦的湿热郁积更为明显。下焦湿热重者可见小便色黄。本舌象常见于现代医学的慢性消化道疾病,如胃炎、十二指肠溃疡、结肠炎,以及慢性泌尿系感染和前列腺炎等,中医辨证为脾肾两虚,内有积滞。

【治疗】法当益脾肾,化郁滞。方用四君子汤和二妙散。

【针刺取穴】中脘、天枢、气海、中极、太溪、足三里、丰隆。

19. The Dim and Pale Tongue with Yellow and Gray Fur at the Root(Figure 7.19)

【Manifestations】The tongue is pale and dim, presenting some red dots at the tip. The coating shows yellow, sticky and dark gray at the root.

【Indications】It results from deficient spleen and kidney as well as internal stagnancy. The yellow coating means heat, while sticky coating means dampness, phlegm or indigested food stagnancy. Therefore the yellow and sticky coating is often related with phlegm and dampness heat pathogen, or stagnant heat from indigested food. For deficient spleen and kidney can cause dysfunction of water metabolism, leading to stagnancy of water dampness in the interior. As a result, dampness heat is obviously stagnated in the lower-jiao, marked by yellow urine. This kind of tongue often occurs in chronic diseases of digestive system, such as gastritis, duodenum ulcer, colonitis, as well as chronic infection of urinary system and prostatitis, which are differentiated by TCM as the syndrome of deficient spleen and kidney combined with stagnancy in the interior.

【Treatment】The therapeutic method should be reinforcing

the spleen and kidney as well as resolving stagnancy. Si-Jun-Zi-Tang(四君子汤) and Er-Miao-San(二妙散) can be taken.

【Selection of acupoints】 Zhongwan (Ren12), Tianshu (St25), Qihai (Ren6), Zhongji (Ren3), Taixi (K3), Zusanli (St36), Fenglong (St40).

第 8 章 淡红舌

1. **淡红红点舌,薄白苔(图 8.1)**

【舌象】舌质淡红,舌的边尖部有许多小红点突出于舌面,舌苔薄白。

【主病】心肝火旺。这张舌象的舌色和舌苔均属正常,不正常之处是舌的边尖部出现的许多红点。红点的形成,中医学认为是脏腑阳气亢盛所致,故主热证。多见于外感热病的极盛期和内伤杂病的脏腑阳热亢盛,常与红舌、绛舌、黄燥苔并见。此舌舌质淡红苔薄白,提示热邪不太重。红点主要分布于舌的边尖部位,所以主病为心肝有热。引起心肝有热的原因很多,较常见的有工作紧张,休息不够;精神焦虑,劳心过度等。

【治法】清泻心肝之火。方剂可用导赤散。

【针刺取穴】内关、神门、少府、大敦、太冲、太溪、三阴交。

Chapter 8 The Light Red Tongue

1. The Reddish Tongue with Red Dots, Covered by Thin White Fur(Figure 8.1)

【Manifestations】 The tongue is light red with many tiny red spots standing out on the sides and tip. The coating is thin and white.

【Indications】 It indicates hyperactive fire of the heart and liver. This tongue picture is normal in color and the coating, but it is abnormal about many red spots on its sides and tip. The reason for that, in TCM opinion, is due to hyperactivity of the viscera Yang, so it reflects heat syndrome. It is usually seen in excessive period of febrile disease, as well as in the disease of the internal injury when Yang heat is hyperactive within the viscera. Usually it is present together with red tongue or crimson tongue, and yellow dry coating. This tongue shows light red color and thin white coating, suggesting less hyperactivity of heat pathogen. The red spots are distributed mainly on the sides and tip, indicating heat in the heart and liver. The reasons of that may be working tensely, shortness of rest, spirit anxiety, and over thinking, etc.

【Treatment】To clear away fire of the heart and liver. The prescription may be Dao-Chi-San(导赤散).

【Selection of acupoints】Neiguan(P6), Shenmen(H7), Shaofu(H8), Dadun(Liv1), Taichong(Liv3), Taixi(K3), Sanyinjiao(Sp6).

2. 淡红齿痕舌,薄白苔(图 8.2)

【舌象】舌质淡红,边缘有牙齿的压痕,舌苔薄白。

【主病】气虚。这张舌象照片基本上可说是正常舌象,即淡红舌薄白苔,不正常的地方在于舌边部的“齿痕”。什么叫齿痕呢,为什么会出现这种现象呢?中医学认为出现这种舌象的原因主要是“气虚”,即人体中属阳的一些物质虚少不足,使舌体中血脉的张力减弱,血、津等物质流行迟缓,这样舌体的弹性就差,遇到牙齿这样的硬物就会被压上模痕而出现齿痕,所以齿痕舌多见于阳气虚的证候。此舌常见于一些身体虚弱的人。

【治疗】补益气血。方用八珍汤。

【针刺取穴】气海、关元、中脘、天枢、足三里、阳陵泉、三阴交、血海。

2. The Reddish Tongue with Tooth-Prints Covered by Thin White Fur(Figure 8.2)

【Manifestations】This is light red tongue, some tooth traces existing on the edges. The coating is thin and white.

【Indications】It indicates Qi deficiency. Generally speaking, the picture as above is normal, i.e. light red tongue and thin white coating. But it is abnormal with some tooth traces on the edges of tongue. In TCM opinion, the main reason for the tongue is Qi deficiency. In other words, some substance of Yang is insufficient. It leads to the blood vessels of the tongue less flexibility, and then causes retarded flow of blood or fluid.

So the tongue body is not elastic, easy to be marked by some tooth traces when it touches hard teeth. Thus the tongue with tooth traces is usually seen in the syndrome of Yang deficiency, mostly occurring in some debility cases.

【Treatment】 To benefit Qi and replenish blood. Ba-Zhen-Tang(八珍汤) can be used.

【Selection of acupoints】 Qihai(Ren6), Guanyuan(Ren4), Zhongwan (Ren12), Tianshu (St25), Zusanli (St36), Yanglingquan(GB34), Sanyinjiao(Sp6), Xuehai(Sp10).

3. 淡红胖嫩舌,薄白干苔(图8.3)

【舌象】舌质淡红,舌体较正常人胖大,舌质纹理细腻。苔质薄而少津,苔色白。

【主病】虚人外感温热病邪,津液受伤。舌质淡红而胖嫩,多见于气虚之人。若感受风热或温热邪气,热伤津液,则舌苔干而少津。邪气在表,尚未入里,故舌色与苔色正常。见于外感病的初起阶段,可出现头痛欲裂,小便黄,脉浮数等症。常见于老年人或体弱之人春季感冒、急性扁桃体炎等病初起之时。

【治疗】辛凉解表,方用银翘散。

【针刺取穴】少商、列缺、合谷、曲池、大椎、风池、足三里、三阴交、阴陵泉。

3. The Reddish, Enlarged and Tender Tongue, Covered by Thin, White and Dry Fur(Figure 8.3)

【Manifestations】 The tongue color is light red and its body is larger than normal one, the texture of the tongue showing fine. The coating is thin and with less moisture, showing white.

【Indications】 It results from the debility constitution with impairment of body fluid by exogenous warm heat pathogens. The tongue marked by light red, puffy and tender is usually seen in the syndrome of Qi deficiency. When invaded by wind heat or warm heat pathogens, the tongue will present dry and less moisture as a result of body fluid damaged. Since the pathogen attacks the exterior and hasn't invaded the interior, the colors of tongue body and tongue coating are still as usual. The tongue can occur at the early stage of the exogenous disease, with symptoms of headache, yellow urine, floating and rapid pulse. It is usually seen in the case of aged people or debility body suffering from flu in spring or acute onset of tonsillitis.

【Treatment】 To relieve the exterior syndrome with acrid and cool herbs. Yin-Qiao-San(银翘散) is commonly applied.

【Selection of acupoints】 Shaoshang (Lu11), Lieque (Lu7), Quchi(LI11), Dazhui(Du14), Fengchi(GB20), Zusanli (St36), Sanyinjiao(Sp6), Yinlingquan(Sp9).

4. 淡红裂纹舌,透明苔(图 8.4)

【舌象】舌质淡红,上有裂纹。苔薄白而透明,因其舌苔极薄,附着在舌面,似苔非苔,所以称为透明苔。

【主病】气阴两伤。舌苔由胃气所生,古人云"胃蒸脾湿上潮而生",因此舌苔的有无反映了胃气和津液的有无存亡。舌上出现裂纹,是阴液不足以濡润之象。由此本舌象提示体内气阴不足,为虚证属内伤病。临床常见植物神经功能紊乱性低热、慢性感染性疾病、内分泌疾病、结核病所引起的发热,以及神经衰弱的病人。中医辨证则属气阴两虚者。

【治疗】补气养阴,用补中益气汤。

【针刺取穴】关元、气海、中脘、天枢、太溪、照海、足三里、三阴交。

4. The Reddish Tongue with Fissures, Covered by transparent Fur(Figure 8.4)

【Manifestations】 The tongue is light red, showing some fissures. The coating is thin, white and transparent. Since it is very thin and attached to the surface, it seems as no coating, and then it is termed transparent coating.

【Indications】 It denotes impairment of both Qi and Yin. For the tongue, coating is formed under the stomach Qi. According to TCM, an upward steaming action of the spleen fluid by the stomach Qi can bring about the tongue coating. So whether existence of the coating or not, reflects the conditions of stomach Qi as well as body fluid. Therefore, fissures on the tongue are the manifestation of insufficient Yin fluid failing in moistening. Thus the picture suggests the syndrome of Qi and Yin deficiency, which belongs to internal injury diseases. It is usually seen in those patients with fever due to dysfunction of vegetative nerve, chronic infectious diseases, endocrine diseases, or tuberculosis, as well as in neurasthenia patients. All diseases as above, differentiated by TCM, are the syndrome of Qi and Yin deficiency.

【Treatment】 To benefit both Qi and nourish Yin. Bu-Zhong-Yi-Qi-Tang(补中益气汤) can be chosen.

【Selection of acupoints】Guanyuan(Ren4), Qihai(Ren6), Zhongwan(Ren12), Tianshu(St25), Taixi(K3), Zhaohai(K6), Zusanli(St36), Sanyinjiao(Sp6).

5. 淡红齿痕舌，白腻湿润苔(图 8.5)

【舌象】舌质淡红,偏暗而有齿痕,苔白腻湿润。

【主病】脾气虚弱,水湿阻滞。这种舌象多因平素脾气不足,脾失健运,而水湿内停所致。此舌象舌质淡红,苔仍属薄白苔本为正常舌象,但其淡红舌中偏紫为平时吸烟过多所致,舌体有齿痕,苔湿滑为脾虚水停之象。临床多见于慢性消化道疾病、肝胆疾病、肺气肿、慢性气管炎、风湿病或各种关节疼痛性病变。

【治疗】健脾利湿。方用参苓白术散加减。

【针刺取穴】阳陵泉、足三里、阴陵泉、三阴交、脾俞、胃俞、肝俞。

5. The Reddish and Tooth Trace Tongue Covered by White, Sticky and Moist Fur(Figure 8.5)

【Manifestations】 The tongue is light red, dark and with tooth traces. The coating is white, sticky and moist.

【Indications】 It results from deficient spleen and dampness retention. This kind of tongue picture is mainly due the deficient spleen that is dysfunction in transforming and transporting, leading to retention of water dampness. The tongue is light red with the thin and white coating, belonging to a normal tongue picture. But its darkness is a sign of over smoking in usual time. The tooth traces and moist coating are the manifestation of deficient spleen with dampness retention. Clinically, it can be seen in chronic diseases of digestive system, liver and gallbladder disorders, emphysema, chronic tracheitis, rheumatism, or painful diseases of the joints.

【Treatment】 To invigorate the spleen and excrete dampness. Modified Shen-Ling-Bai-Zhu-San(参苓白术散) should be chosen.

【Selection of acupoints】Yanglingquan (GB34), Zusanli (St36), Yinlingquan(Sp9), Sanyinjiao(Sp6), Pishu(UB20), Weishu(UB21), Ganshu(UB18).

6. 淡红偏暗舌,白腐苔(图 8.6)

【舌象】 舌质淡红偏暗,舌苔白腐。

【主病】 食积痰浊,内蕴肠胃。腐苔是因体内有食、痰停滞,而阳热有余,蒸腾胃腐浊之气上泛而成。若腐苔揩之即去,为正气驱邪外出。舌质偏暗,为痰食阻滞,气血运行不畅之象。或见胸胁作痛,咯吐脓痰量多。可见于消化不良、胃炎或肺脓疡等病症。

【治疗】 食积者治以消积导滞,方用保和丸,以黄连煎汤送服。

【针刺取穴】合谷、太冲、血海、三阴交、足三里、条口、阳陵泉、中脘、天枢。

6. The Reddish and Dim Tongue with White and Curdy Fur(Figure 8.6)

【Manifestations】 The tongue is light red and dark. The coating is white and curdy.

【Indications】 It indicates indigested food and phlegm turbidity stagnating in the gastrointestinal tract. The curdy coating is produced by curdy turbid pathogen in the stomach, which ascends to the surface of tongue under an upwards steaming action of excessive Yang. If the curdy coating is easy to be wiped out, it means pathogen expelled by vital Qi. The dark tongue is a sign of unsmooth flow of Qi and blood because of phlegm and food retention. The symptoms associated with the tongue may be pain in the chest and hypochondrium, expectorating profuse thick sputum. The tongue picture as above can be seen in dyspepsia, gastritis, or lung abscess, etc.

【Treatment】 The method is to remove stagnant food for the syndrome of food retention. Bao-He-Wan(保和丸) can be used, which should be taken with Huang-Lian-Tang(黄连汤) together.

【Selection of acupoints】Hegu(LI4), Taichong(Liv3), Xuehai(Sp10), Sanyinjiao(Sp6), Zusanli(St36), Yanglingquan(GB34), Zhongwan(Ren12), Tianshu(St25).

7. 淡红齿痕舌,薄白腻苔(图 8.7)

【舌象】舌质淡红,边有齿痕,苔薄白腻。

【主病】脾虚停湿。舌质淡红为正常舌象,但其舌边有齿痕,苔薄白而腻,说明脾气虚弱、水湿内聚或外感寒湿。湿邪困阻之证。临床常见心功能不全、肾功能衰竭,以及各种消化系统慢性疾病,如胃炎、肠炎、肠结核等病变。

【治疗】以健脾益气、芳香化湿为主。①外感寒湿者可用羌活胜湿汤加减;②湿阻上焦可用胜湿汤加减;③湿阻中焦者可用胃苓汤加减;④脾虚湿困药用加味异功散。

【针刺取穴】三阴交、阴陵泉、足三里、条口、关元、气海、中脘、天枢。

7. The Reddish Tongue with Tooth Traces, Covered by Thin, White and Sticky Fur(Figure 8.7)

【Manifestations】 The tongue is light red and marked by tooth traces. The coating is thin, white and sticky.

【Indications】 It indicates deficient spleen with dampness retention. The light red tongue is normal, but those tooth traces as well as sticky coating are abnormal, suggesting the spleen insufficiency with water dampness stagnation, or with exogenous cold dampness invasion. It is the syndrome of dampness obstruction, clinically seen in the cases of cardiac insufficiency, renal failure, as well as the chronic diseases of digestive system, such as gastritis, enteritis, tuberculosis of intestine, etc.

【Treatment】 The treatment is mainly to invigorate the spleen and benefit Qi, as well as to resolve dampness with fragrant medicine. (1) Modified Qiang-Huo-Sheng-Shi-Tang(羌活胜湿汤) can be used for the exterior syndrome of cold dampness; (2) Modified Sheng-Shi-Tang(胜湿汤) can treat dampness obstruction in the up-jiao; (3) Modified Wei-Ling-Tang (胃苓汤) should be applied for dampness obstruction in the middle-jiao; (4) Jia-Wei-Yi-Gong-San(加味异功散) is suitable for deficient spleen with dampness accumulation.

【Selection of acupoints】 Sanyinjiao(Sp6), Yinlingquan (Sp9), Zusanli (St36), Guanyuan (Ren4), Qihai (Ren6), Zhongwan(Ren12), Tianshu(St25).

8. 淡红红点舌,白腐苔(图 8.8)

【舌象】舌质淡暗红而偏胖,舌尖有红点,舌中部苔白腐。

【主病】气虚血瘀痰凝。这种舌象多因久病心肺气虚血瘀,痰湿停滞所致。舌质淡而偏胖为心气虚,舌暗红为心血痹阻,舌尖有红点为血郁痰郁化热之象,苔白腐为痰湿内盛所致。唇甲青紫,倦怠,食欲不振,大便不调,脉缓无力或结代。临床可见于冠心病,肺心病等各种心肺之脏的慢性病变。

【治疗】益气活血,兼祛痰湿。方用生脉饮加味。

【针刺取穴】足三里、阴陵泉、三阴交、条口、合谷、太冲、血海。

8. The Reddish Tongue with Red Spots, Covered by White and Curdy Fur(Figure 8.8)

【Manifestations】 The tongue is light red and dark, being enlarged, showing red spots on the tip. The coating is white and curdy especially in the middle.

【Indications】 It demotes Qi deficiency and blood stasis, as well as phlegm retention. This kind of tongue is usually caused by prolonged disease of Qi deficiency of the heart and lung, complicated with blood stasis and phlegm dampness retention. The tongue being pale and enlarged is the result of the heart Qi deficiency, while the dark red tongue is manifestation of the heart blood stasis. Those red spots on the tip indicate heat tendency transformed from stagnant blood and phlegm. The curdy coating results from excessive phlegm dampness. In such conditions, the symptoms, such as blue purplish lips and nails, lassitude, poor appetite, abnormal stools, slow and weak pulses, or knotted and intermittent pulse, are frequently seen, which usually occur in some chronic diseases of the heart and lung, such as coronary heart disease, pulmonary heart disease, etc.

【Treatment】The treatment method should be to strengthen Qi and promote blood circulation, as well as to eliminate phlegm dampness. Modified Sheng-Mai-Yin(生脉饮) can be chosen.

【Selection of acupoints】Zusanli (St36), Yinlingquan (Sp9), Sanyinjiao(Sp6), Tiaokou(St36), Hegu(LI4), Taichong (Liv3), Xuehai(Sp10).

9. 淡红裂纹齿痕舌，中部淡黄苔(图 8.9)

【舌象】舌质淡红，舌体胖嫩，上有裂纹，边有齿痕，舌中部苔薄黄。

【主病】脾气虚损，湿邪内停。舌体浮胖娇嫩为虚证，边有齿痕而又有裂纹，说明体内脾气运化水湿的功能减弱，湿邪内生。湿邪停滞可郁而化热，上蒸于舌，舌苔见淡黄。中部苔黄，说明病位在中焦脾胃。此舌象提示患者常为脾胃气虚，湿邪内停化热之症。食无味，口不渴或渴不欲饮，大便溏泻，小便不利，脉象虚大。本舌象常见于现代医学的慢性胃功能紊乱、消化不良、高血压、慢性肾盂肾炎，中医辨证为脾胃气虚，湿邪内停。

【治疗】健脾利湿。药用参苓白术散。

【针刺取穴】足三里、三阴交、阴陵泉、合谷、曲池、脾俞、胃俞 、肝俞。

9. The Reddish Tongue Marked by Tooth Prints and Fissures, Covered with The Light Yellow and Sticky Fur in The Center(Figure 8.9)

【Manifestations】The tongue is light red with its body enlarged, showing fissures on the surface and tooth traces at the edges. The coating in the middle is thin and yellow.

【Indications】It means deficient spleen Qi and dampness retention. The body of tongue being puffy and tender indicates deficiency syndrome. Marked by tooth traces and fissures, the tongue picture is a result of dampness retention due to dysfunction of the spleen, which fails to transform and transport water dampness. Dampness retention can change into heat that can be learnt through light yellow color of the coating. Since the yellow coating is obvious in the center of the tongue, it means the disease is located in the middle-jiao. Therefore the picture of tongue suggests that this is a syndrome of deficient spleen with dampness heat transformed from retention. The symptoms, such as tasteless sensation of food, no thirst, or thirst without desire for drinking, loose stool, dysuria, weak and large pulse, can be seen. The tongue picture as above often occurs in diseases, such as chronic dysfunction of the stomach, dyspepsia, hypertension, chronic pyelonephritis, which are differentiated by TCM as deficient spleen with dampness retention.

【Treatment】 The treatment should be reinforcing the spleen and excreting dampness. Shen-Ling-Bai-Zhu-San(参苓白术散) can be chosen.

【Selection of acupoints】Zusanli(St36), Sanyinjiao(Sp6), Yinlingquan(Sp9), Hegu(LI4), Quchi(LI11), Pishu(UB20), Weishu(UB21), Ganshu(UB18).

10. 淡红舌,白腐淡黄苔(图 8.10)

【舌象】舌质淡红,苔白腐,中部微黄。

【主病】痰湿内停,郁而化热,苔质腐为体内停有湿热或痰浊,脾失健运之象。湿浊郁久化热,故苔色由白而渐转黄。舌质淡红,表明虽有痰湿停于体内,但正气未伤,属于新病、轻病。质粘或大便泄泻不爽。可见于消化系统和呼吸系统的急性感染,如消化不良、胃肠炎、气管炎、哮喘及感冒、流行性感冒并发感染者。

【治疗】(1)湿邪入里化热,热象明显者,可用白虎加苍术汤为主治疗。(2)若感受暑湿邪气,头胀、胸闷泛恶者,可用藿香正气散。(3)脾胃湿热者可用清热化湿的方法,药用连朴饮。(4)肺有痰热者可用清肺热化痰浊之法。

【针刺取穴】天枢、中脘、足三里、丰隆、阳陵泉、三阴交。

10. The Reddish Tongue Covered with Curdy White and

Yellow Fur(Figure 8.10)

【Manifestations】The tongue is light red. The coating is curdy and white but shows light yellow in the middle.

【Indications】It suggests dampness retention transforming into heat. The curdy coating is a manifestation of dampness heat or dampness turbidity stagnating in the interior due to the spleen dysfunction in transformation. Dampness turbidity can change into heat if it is stagnant for a period, which can be known through the change of coating color from white to yellow. The light red of the tongue is the sign of vital Qi uninjured although there is dampness turbidity stagnating insides. It is still a new disease, and mild illness. Unsmooth stools may be seen linked to this tongue picture. It usually appears in diseases of digestive system, respiratory system, complicated with acute infection, such as dyspepsia, gastroenteritis, tracheitis, asthma, or catch cold, and flu in a combination with infection.

【Treatment】(1) Bai-Hu-Jia-Cang-Zhu-Tang(白虎加苍术汤) can be used for the interior heat transformed from exterior dampness. (2) Huo-Xiang-Zheng-Qi-San(藿香正气散) can be tried for the invasion of summer heat and dampness pathogen. (3) Lian-Po-Yin(连朴饮) can be chosen for the dampness heat in the spleen and stomach. (4) It is a suitable method to eliminate phlegm turbidity and clear away the lung heat for the phlegm heat in the lung.

【Selection of acupoints】Tianshu (St25), Zhongwan (Ren12), Zusanli (St36), Fenglong (St40), Yanglingquan (GB34), Sanyinjiao(Sp6).

11. 淡红红点舌,薄黄苔(图 8.11)

【舌象】舌质淡红,夹有红点,舌边有齿痕,苔薄黄。

【主病】风热侵犯肺胃。这种舌象见于素体脾胃气虚又感受风热病邪。舌质淡红夹红点,在舌尖部较多,为肺热壅盛。舌中部苔薄黄为胃热初起,舌边有齿痕为素体脾虚之象。临床可见各种急性感染性疾病,如气管炎、感冒或扁桃腺炎,或慢性胃炎、胆囊炎、肝炎、胰腺炎等病变的急性发作,为病情较轻的表现。

【治疗】清泻肺胃之热。方用黄连解毒汤加减。

【针刺取穴】合谷、曲池、足三里、太渊 、尺泽、少商。

11. The Reddish Tongue with Red Spots, Covered by Thin and Yellow Fur(Figure 8.11)

【Manifestations】 The tongue is light red with some red spots, tooth traces at edges. The coating is thin and yellow.

【Indications】 It indicates the invasion of the lung and stomach by pathogenic wind heat. It is usually seen in the case of deficient spleen Qi affected by wind heat pathogen. The tongue is light red with some obvious red spots on the tip, meaning excessive heat in the lung. The yellow color presenting in the middle of the tongue is a sign of the stomach heat newly arising. The tooth traces on the sides of tongue are caused by constitutional deficient spleen. This kind of the tongue picture can be seen in many acute infective diseases, such as tracheitis, flu, tonsillitis, or acute onset of chronic gastritis, cholecystitis, hepatitis, pancreatitis, etc. It is a manifestation of mild diseases.

【Treatment】 The treatment is to clear away heat of the lung and stomach. The prescription is modified Huang-Lian-Jie-Du-Tang(黄连解毒汤).

【Selection of acupoints】Hegu(LI4), Quchi(LI11), Zusanli (St36), Taiyuan(Lu9), Chize(Lu5), Shaoshang(Lu11).

12. **淡红偏暗舌,黄腻苔(图** 8.12)

【舌象】舌质淡红偏暗,舌尖红,苔黄腻。

【主病】风热表证或风寒化热入里。外感病初起,病情轻浅,尚未伤及气血及内脏,故舌质可仍保持正常的淡红色。随着年龄的增长,舌质在淡红的基础上略偏暗,可不作病色论。舌苔薄黄,提示感受的是风热邪气或风寒邪气入里化热。因苔质尚未由薄转厚,标志着邪热不甚、入里未深。欲饮,咽喉肿痛。常见于流行性感冒、气管炎等上呼吸道感染。

【治疗】以发热、头痛、咽喉肿痛的风热表证为主者,治宜清解表热,方用银翘散。

【针刺取穴】大椎、风池、合谷、曲池、少商、列缺、足三里、丰隆。

12. The Reddish and Dim Tongue with Yellow and Sticky Fur(Figure 8.12)

【Manifestations】The tongue is light red and dark, the tip is red. The coating is yellow and sticky.

【Indications】It indicates the exterior syndrome of wind heat, or wind cold pathogen changing into the interior heat. When the exogenous disease begins, its pathogenic condition is mild, and hasn't affected the viscera or Qi and blood, so it can keep the tongue as normal as light red color. The light red color can grow to light dark along with ages, which shouldn't be considered the illness color. The thin and yellow coating means that the invasion of pathogen is wind-heat, or wind-cold, which has changed into interior heat. The pathogenic heat is not strong enough to invade deeply. The coating is thin and not yet thick. The tongue picture is often marked by symptoms of sore throat, and liking to drink, etc. Therefore it is often seen in respiratory tract diseases such as flu, tracheitis, and so on.

【Treatment】The treatment should be relieving the exterior syndrome and clearing away heat. Yin-Qiao-San(银翘散) can be used.

【Selection of acupoints】Dazhui(Du14), Fengchi(GB20), Hegu(LI4), Quchi(LI11), Shaoshang(Lu11), Lieque(Lu7), Zusanli(St36), Fenglong(St40).

13. 淡红瘀斑瘀点舌,薄黄腻苔(图 8.13)

【舌象】舌质淡红,边有淡紫瘀斑和暗红瘀点。舌苔薄腻淡黄而润。

【主病】气滞血瘀,血热瘀滞。舌边属肝胆,肝郁气滞,气滞血瘀,故舌边见淡紫瘀斑。郁而化火,故舌苔淡黄。血分蕴热,故见暗红点,热未伤津,故苔腻而润。常见于消化道疾病,如慢性胃肠炎、溃疡病、胃神经官能症、肝炎、胆囊炎、胆石症等。可有胸胁脘腹胀痛或刺痛,忧思恼怒等情绪波动可使病势加重,痛点常固定拒按,常嗳气泛酸或呕血、便血、口苦、心烦、失眠。

【治疗】宜用理气活血清热法。方用柴胡疏肝饮合失笑散加减。

【针刺取穴】太冲、合谷、阳陵泉、足三里、足临泣、中脘、天枢 。

13. The Reddish Tongue with Petechia Covered by Thin, Yellow and Sticky Fur(Figure 8.13)

【Manifestations】 The tongue is light red with some purplish spots and dark red dots at the edges. The coating is thin, sticky and yellowish with moisture.

【Indications】 It results from Qi stagnation and blood stasis as well as stagnant blood heat. Since the edges of the tongue correspond to the liver and gallbladder, the petechia appearing at the edges indicate the liver Qi stagnancy and blood stasis. Stagnation transforms into heat, so it gives rise to the yellowish coating. The dark red dots on the tongue suggest pathogenic heat stagnated in the blood system, while moist and sticky coating means body fluid uninjured by heat. It is seen in the diseases of digestive tract, such as chronic gastroenteritis, ulcer, gastroneurosis, hepatitis, cholecystitis, gallstone, marked by distending pain or stabbing pain over chest and hypochondrium, or epigastrium and abdomen, which are usually aggravated by intensely emotional changes. The pain is fixed and aversion to palpation, often accompanied with belching, acid regurgitation, or vomiting blood, bloody stools, bitter taste in the mouth, restlessness, insomnia and so on.

【Treatment】 The method is to regulate Qi and promote blood circulation as well as to clear away heat. Modified Chai-Hu-Shu-Gan-Yin(柴胡疏肝饮) with Shi-Xiao-San(失笑散) can be tried.

【Selection of acupoints】Taichong(Liv3), Hegu(LI4), Yanglingquan(GB34), Zusanli(St36), Zulinqi(GB41), Zhongwan (Ren12), Tianshu(St25) .

14. 淡红舌,根黄腻苔(图 8.14)

【舌象】 舌质淡红,有红点;苔质腻,苔色白,根部黄。

【主病】 食积或湿邪困脾,郁而化热。淡红舌为正常舌质。病而舌质未见异常,表明为新病或轻病,尚未影响人体的脏腑气血。苔质腻说明感受的邪气性质为湿。苔色白而根部黄,说明邪气有化热之象。

【治疗】伤于饮食,食积内停者,治以消导和胃,可用保和丸。

【针刺取穴】中脘、天枢、足三里、阳陵泉、三阴交、丰隆。

14. The Reddish Tongue with Yellow and Sticky Fur(Figure 8.14)

【Manifestations】 The tongue is light red with some red dots. The coating is sticky and white, its root is yellowish.

【Indications】 It is due to food retention or obstruction of the spleen by dampness, which has transformed into heat. In TCM opinion, the tongue being light red is normal in color. If it is seen in pathogenic condition, it means a new illness or mild disease when the viscera and Qi-blood haven't been affected. The sticky coating indicates the pathogen suffered from belonging to dampness. The coating is whiteness but yellow at the root, suggesting a heat tendency transformed from stagnation.

【Treatment】 The treatment should be removing food retention and promoting digestion for the syndrome of food retention. Bao-He-Wan(保和丸) is a property choice.

【Selection of acupoints】Zhongwan (Ren12), Tianshu (St25), Zusanli (St36), Yanglingquan (GB34), Sanyinjiao (Sp6), Fenglong(St40).

15. 淡红红点舌,白腻淡黄苔(图 8.15)

【舌象】舌质淡红,略显齿痕而稍胖,舌尖有很多红点。舌苔白腻,中根部较厚,已显淡黄。

【主病】脾虚湿盛,湿郁化热。齿痕舌白腻苔是脾虚湿盛之证;湿邪内蕴,郁久化热,故苔转淡黄,尖生红点。该舌象常见于胃肠、肝胆等消化系统疾患,如慢性胃肠炎、肝炎、胆囊炎等,以及妇女慢性盆腔炎。症见脘腹或胁肋胀痛,胸闷恶心,呕吐酸水。

【治疗】法当益气健脾,化湿清热。方用参苓白术散合栀子柏皮汤加减。

【针刺取穴】足三里、阴陵泉、三阴交、太冲、天枢、中脘。

15. The Reddish Tongue with Red Dots, Covered by White, Sticky and Yellowish Fur(Figure 8.15)

【Manifestations】 The tongue is light red and slightly enlarged with tooth traces. There are many red dots at the tongue tip. The coating is white and sticky, it is thick and yellowish in its center.

【Indications】 It reflects the deficient spleen and excessive dampness that has changed into heat. The tooth-marked tongue with sticky white coating is a manifestation of the spleen deficiency with excessive dampness. Prolonged stagnancy of dampness can transform into heat so that the coating turns to yellowish and generates some red dots at the tip. The picture of the tongue often occurs in diseases of the gastrointestinal system and the liver-gallbladder system, such as chronic gastroenteritis, hepatitis, cholecystitis, as well as chronic pelvic inflammation of women. The symptoms liked with the tongue may be distending pain in epigastrium and abdomen, or in hypochondrium and rib region, stuffiness of chest, nausea, vomiting acid liquid, and so on.

【Treatment】 The method should be to benefit Qi and reinforce the spleen, as well as to resolve dampness and clear away heat. Modified Shen-Ling-Bai-Zhu-San(参苓白术散) with Zhi-Zi-Bai-Pi-Tang(栀子柏皮汤) can be chosen.

【Selection of acupoints】Zusanli (St36), Yinlingquan (Sp9), Sanyinjiao (Sp6), Taichong (Liv3), Tianshu (St25), Zhongwan (Ren12).

16. 淡红尖红舌，淡黄干苔(图 8.16)

【舌象】 舌质淡红，舌尖红赤，苔淡黄略腻而干。

【主病】 里热初起。这种舌象常见外感风寒或风热之邪，外邪入里化热之开始阶段。舌质本为淡红属正常舌象。舌尖红赤有许多红点为外邪犯肺，肺热始盛之象。苔淡黄也属外邪化热未尽之象，舌中根部有腻苔为病人原有脾虚湿蕴或食积的表现。临床可见急性上呼吸道感染，流行性感冒，急性扁桃腺炎，某些传染病的初期，如腮腺炎、流行性脑膜炎、麻疹的初期。

【治疗】清热解表，润肺化浊。方用银翘散加减。

【针刺取穴】少商、鱼际、列缺、合谷、曲池、大椎、风池。

16. The Reddish Tongue with Red Tip Covered by Yellowish and Dry Fur(Figure 8.16)

【Manifestations】 The tongue is reddish with its tip reddened. The coating is yellowish, lightly sticky and dry.

【Indications】 It suggests interior heat arising. The tongue picture is usually seen at the early stage of interior heat transformed from exogenous pathogen of wind-cold or wind-heat. The reddish tongue is a normal picture, but many red dots at the tip suggest the lung heat tending to excess after the lung invaded by exogenous pathogen. The coating being yellowish means the interior heat arising but the exterior pathogen not disappearing. The tongue shows sticky coating in the middle and at the root as a result of stagnant dampness or food retention due to spleen deficiency previously. This kind of tongue pictures can be seen in many diseases, for instance, acute infection of upper respiratory tract, flu, acute tonsillitis, as well as in early days of some epidemics, such as parotitis, epidemic meningitis, measles, and so on.

【Treatment】 The treatment should be relieving the exterior syndrome and clearing away heat, as well as nourishing the lung and resolving turbidity. Modified Yin-Qiao-San(银翘散) can be chosen.

【Selection of acupoints】Shaoshang(Lu11), Yuji(Lu10), Lieque(Lu7), Hegu (LI4), Quchi (LI11), Dazhui (Du14), Fengchi(GB20).

第9章 红舌

1. 红光莹裂纹舌(图 9.1)

【舌象】舌质红有裂纹，中部光莹，两边少许白垢似苔非苔。

【主病】肺胃阴伤。此舌象多见于外感热病高热极期之后，出现的肺胃阴液大伤。外感热病是人体感受外邪而引起急性发热为主的疾病。它包括了现代医学中以高热为主的多种传染病，如流行性脑脊髓膜炎、麻疹、腥红热等。这些疾病在高热极期(如伤寒病的阳明病、温热病的气分证)，都会因热伤津液，而造成肺胃阴液的大量耗损，而出现此种舌象。

【治疗】滋养肺胃津液。方用沙参麦门冬汤。

【针刺取穴】大椎、合谷、曲池、少商、太溪、照海、三阴交、足三里。

Chapter 9 The Red Tongue

1. The Red Glossy Tongue with Fissures(Figure 9.1)

【Manifestations】The tongue is red with fissures, showing glossy in the center. Some white substance seems as the coating on the both sides.

【Indications】The tongue suggests impairment of Yin in the lung and stomach. It is usually seen when the Yin fluid of the lung and stomach has been severe damaged after intensely high fever of exogenous febrile disease. The exogenous febrile disease is the illness marked by acute fever due to invasion of exogenous pathogen. It includes many infectious diseases of modern medicine manifested mainly with high fever, such as epidemic cerebrospinal meningitis, measles, and scarlet fever, etc. All these diseases may present this kind of tongue pictures in the period of intensely high fever (such as Yang-ming syndrome of cold stroke, or Qi-fen syndrome of seasonal febrile diseases), because that pathogenic heat impairs the body fluid and produces exhaustion of Yin fluid.

【Treatment】 The treatment should aim at replenishing body fluid of the lung and stomach. Sha-Shen-Mai-Dong-Tang (沙参麦冬汤) is a proper choice.

【Selection of acupoints】 Dazhui (Du14), Hegu (LI4), Quchi (LI11), Shaoshang (Lu11), Taixi (K3), Zhaohai (K6), Sanyinjiao (Sp6), Zusanli (St36).

2. 红嫩无苔舌(图9.2)

【舌象】舌质红,舌面无苔,望之似有光泽,但扪之却十分干燥,质地不苍老反见娇嫩。

【主病】胃阴大伤或胃阴亡失。《辨舌指南》指出:"若舌绛而光亮者,胃阴亡也。"此舌象外感病主要见于温热病后期,热灼胃津致胃阴大伤甚则胃阴亡失,内伤病多见于一些慢性消耗性疾病的晚期,如癌症晚期、肝硬化失代偿出现腹水后,以及结核病、心脑血管病的重症等。临床见此舌象,提示胃阴大伤,病情危重。

【治疗】补益胃阴。方用一贯煎。

【针刺取穴】足三里、三阴交、阴陵泉、太溪、照海、脾俞、胃俞。

2. The Red and Tender Tongue without Fur (Figure 9.2)

【Manifestations】 The tongue is red without coating, looking glossy. It feels very dry. The property isn't rough but tender.

【Indications】 It means heavy impairment or exhaustion of the stomach Yin. It is pointed out in an ancient book "Guiding For The Tongue Differentiation" that the glossy tongue reflects exhaustion of the stomach Yin. In exogenous disease, this kind of tongues is mainly seen at the late stage of seasonal febrile diseases when the stomach Yin has been severely consumed or even exhausted by heat pathogen. In internal injury diseases, it is usually present at the advanced stage of some chronic consumptive illness, such as cancer, ascites due to decompensation of hepatocirrhosis, as well as severe cases of tuberculosis, cardiac cerebral vascular disease, and so on. In clinic, the tongue picture suggests critical condition with heavily consumed stomach Yin.

【Treatment】 The method of replenishing stomach yin should be adopted. Yi-Guan-Jian(一贯煎) is a suitable prescription.

【Selection of acupoints】Zusanli(St36), Sanyinjiao(Sp6), Yinlingquan(Sp9), Taixi(K3), Zhaohai(K6), Pishu(UB20), Weishu(UB21).

3. 红瘦裂纹舌少苔(图 9.3)

【舌象】舌质红,舌形较瘦有裂纹,苔少。

【主病】阴虚阳亢。此舌为一肝阴虚阳亢,以眩晕(高血压)为主症的患者的舌象照片。年老肝肾阴精化生不足,不足以涵敛肝阳,所以阳气亢于上,可见舌质红。这种病证的根本是阴精不足,所以舌体失充而现瘦薄有裂纹,阴虚无以养苔,故苔少或无苔。

【治疗】平肝潜阳。方药可用天麻钩藤饮。

【针刺取穴】列缺、照海、太溪、太冲、行间、四神冲、风池。

3. The Red and Thin Tongue with Fissures and less coating(Figure 9.3)

【Manifestations】 The tongue is red and emaciated, marked by fissures on the surface. The coating is less.

【Indications】 It means hyperactivity Yang due to deficient Yin. This tongue photo taken from a patient with dizziness complaint (hypertension) that belongs to the syndrome of Yin deficiency and Yang hyperactivity. For the aged people, the Yin essence can not be produced enough to check the liver Yang, and consequently Yang is hyperactive upwards, bringing the tongue red in color. Since the syndrome is basically Yin essence insufficient, the tongue fails to be nourished and supported, leading to the tongue emaciated and fissured, the coating less or no at all.

【Treatment】 The method of soothing the liver and subduing Yang can be applied. Tian-Ma-Gou-Teng-Yin(天麻钩藤

饮）should be tried.

【Selection of acupoints】Lieque（Lu7），Zhaohai（K6），Taixi（K3），Taichong（Liv3），Xingjian（Liv2），Sishenchong（Extra11），Fengchi（GB20）.

4. **红舌少苔（图 9.4）**

【舌象】舌质色红、有裂纹，苔少。

【主病】胃阴虚损。胃为阳土，喜润而恶燥，脾为阴土，喜燥而恶湿，这一脏一腑燥湿相济，阴阳相合，才能完成饮食物的受纳、腐熟、消化、吸收。胃阴虚损常可影响胃受纳腐熟水谷和胃气的和降。此舌象可见于现代医学胃及十二指肠溃疡、慢性胃炎、萎缩性胃炎等疾病。

【治疗】养阴益胃。可选用益胃汤。

【针刺取穴】足三里、阴陵泉、三阴交、脾俞、胃俞、肾俞。

4. The Red Tongue With Less Fur（Figure 9.4）

【Manifestations】The tongue is with red fissures and less coating.

【Indications】It is a sign of the deficient stomach Yin. In TCM opinion, the stomach corresponds to the Yang-earth, being preference for moistness and intolerance to dryness, while the spleen corresponds to the Yin-earth, being preference for dryness and intolerance to moistness. This pair of Zang-Fu organs is harmonious in their natures of dryness and moistness as well as Yin and Yang, so as to complete the process of receiving, soaking, digesting, and assimilating for food. The deficient stomach Yin is able to affect the function of food reception and digestion as well as the downward ability of itself. The picture as above is usually seen in diseases, such as duodenum ulcer, chronic gastritis, atrophic gastritis, etc.

【Treatment】It should be adopted nourishing Yin and benefiting the stomach. Yi-Wei-Tang（益胃汤）may be chosen.

【Selection of acupoints】Zusanli（St36），Yinlingquan（Sp9），Sanyinjiao（Sp6），Pishu（UB20），Weishu（UB21），ShenShu（UB23）.

5. **胖大红点舌少苔（图 9.5）**

【舌象】舌体胖大淡红，边尖部有红点，舌苔极少而薄白。

【主病】气虚风热感冒。舌尖部属上焦心肺，风热邪气初袭人体，部位在皮毛肺卫，所以舌体表现为边尖部红点，在内伤为血分蕴热。此舌为素体气虚者，患风热感冒初起的卫分证舌象。

【治疗】益气清解表热。方用桑菊饮。

【针刺取穴】太渊、列缺、合谷、曲池、大椎、足三里、阴陵泉。

5. The Enlarged Tongue with Red Dots and Less Fur(Figure 9.5)

【Manifestations】 The tongue is enlarged and light red, showing some red dots at the edges and tip. The coating is less, thin and white.

【Indications】 It results from Qi deficiency accompanied with exogenous disease of wind heat. According to TCM, the tongue tip corresponds to the upper-jiao, the lung and heart. Since wind heat and pathogenic factors invade the body originally, they are located in the exterior and the lung-wei system, bringing the sign of red dots on the sides and tongue tip. Occurring in the internal injury disease, the red spots mean stagnant heat in the blood system. This kind of tongues is a manifestation of the debility constitution complicated with the Wei syndrome caused by exogenous wind heat pathogens.

【Treatment】 It should be treated as benefiting Qi, relieving the exterior, and clearing away heat. Sang-Ju-Yin(桑菊饮) is suitable.

【Selection of acupoints】Taiyuan(Lu9), Lieque(Lu7), Hegu(LI4), Quchi(LI11), Dazhui(Du14), Zusanli(St36), Yinlingquan(Sp6).

6. **红舌类剥苔(图9.6)**

【舌象】舌质红有裂纹，类剥苔。

【主病】邪热已退，气阴两伤。这种舌象的产生是由于热邪损伤气阴，舌苔失去气阴的养护曾一度剥落，后正气渐复，又生出了新苔。

【治疗】补益气阴,方药可用三才汤。

【针刺取穴】气海、关元、中脘、足三里、三阴交、列缺、照海。

6. The Red Tongue with Exfoliated Fur(Figure 9.6)

【Manifestations】 The tongue is red and fissured. The coating seems as exfoliated.

【Indications】 It reflects that pathogenic heat has disappeared but Qi and Yin have been damaged. This kind of the tongue coating is formed because of impairment of Qi and Yin by heat pathogen. For the coating fails to be supported and nourished, it may be partly exfoliated for a period. And later, when the vital Qi is restored, it can present the new coating as the picture showing.

【Treatment】 It should be to benefit Qi and replenish Yin. San-Cai-Tang(三才汤) can be tried.

【Selection of acupoints】Qihai(Ren6), Guanyuan(Ren4), Zhongwan(Ren12), Zusanli(St36), Sanyinjiao(Sp6), Lieque (Lu7), Zhaohai(K6).

7. 红夹红点舌少苔(图 9.7)

【舌象】舌质红而有许多红点,苔少。

【主病】热盛阴伤。这种舌象多因外感热邪入里或脏腑热盛,以致阴液耗伤。舌红夹红点为里热炽盛,苔少说明津液已伤,舌边有齿痕为素体脾胃气虚之象。或饥不欲食,大便干燥,小便黄赤,或频数疼痛,脉数。临床可见于慢性胃炎、肾盂肾炎、肺炎恢复期或过敏性紫癜等免疫系统疾病、糖尿病或急性传染病的恢复期。

【治疗】清热滋阴。方用二冬汤加味。

【针刺取穴】大椎、曲池、合谷、内庭、列缺、照海、太溪。

7. The Red Tongue with Red Dots, Covered by Less Fur (Figure 9.7)

【Manifestations】 The tongue is red with some red spots. The coating is less.

【Indications】 It indicates the consumption of Yin by excessive heat. The heat pathogen arises from exogenous heat that invades the interior, or from excessive heat within the Zang-Fu organs. So the tongue showing red and some red spots suggests intense heat of the interior, while the less coating indicates consumption of the body fluid. The tooth traces at the edges are the sign of original deficiency of the spleen and stomach. Symptoms linked with the tongue may be as follows: hungry but without desire for food intake, dry stool, dark yellow urine, or frequent and aching urination, and rapid pulse, etc. Clinically, the tongue can occur in diseases of chronic gastritis, pyelonephritis, pneumonia in its recovery period, or anaphylactoid purpura, or diabetes, or acute epidemical disease during its recovery period, and so on.

【Treatment】 The method should be to clear away heat and nourish Yin. Modified Er-Dong-Tang(二冬汤) can be used.

【Selection of acupoints】Dazhui(Du14), Quchi(LI11), Hegu(LI4), Neiting(St44), Lieque(Lu7), Zhaohai(K6), Taixi(K3).

8. **红嫩舌光剥苔**(图 9.8)

【舌象】舌质红,娇嫩,舌苔光剥。

【主病】阴虚内热。舌色深于正常者为红舌,主热证。但有实热、虚热的不同,舌质的老嫩,是辨别虚实的关键。舌质粗糙、坚敛苍老的,称为"老"舌,主实证、热证。舌质细腻、娇嫩的,称为"嫩"舌,多见于虚证。此舌象舌质红而娇嫩,舌苔光剥,故为阴虚内热证的舌象,此为心阴虚证患者的舌象。

【治疗】滋心阴养心血,安神定志。可选用天王补心丹。

【针刺取穴】中冲、内关、神门、四神冲、列缺、照海、太溪。

8. The Red and Tender Tongue without Fur(Figure 9.8)

【Manifestations】 The tongue is red, showing tender. The coating is all exfoliated.

【Indications】 It is a sign of Yin deficiency due to the internal heat. The tongue being redder than normal is termed red tongue, indicating heat syndromes which include excessive heat and deficient heat. The tender or rough of the tongue is the standard for judging these two types of heat. If the tongue is rough, solid, and tough, it is named "Lao", i.e. old, suggesting excessive syndrome and heat syndrome. If the tongue is fine and tender, it is known as "Nen", i.e. delicate, meaning deficiency syndrome. The picture as above is a red and tender tongue without coating, so it is a manifestation of Yin deficiency with the internal heat. It is taken from a patient of the heart Yin deficiency.

【Treatment】 It should be treated as nourishing the heart Yin and blood, as well as tranquilizing the mind. Tian-Wang-Bu-Xin-Dan(天王补心丹) can be tried.

【Selection of acupoints】Zhongchong(P9), Neiguan(P6), Shenmen(H7), Sishenchong(Extra11), Lieque(Lu7), Zhaohai(K6), Taixi(K3).

9. 红偏暗舌白厚腻苔(图9.9)

【舌象】舌质红,舌苔白腻。

【主病】阴虚夹湿。这种舌象的形成是素有阴亏虚火,又过食肥甘厚味,或过食冷饮冷食所致。原有阴虚,所以舌质偏红,又有湿浊之邪阻遏阳气,故舌苔白腻。

【治疗】散湿和胃。方用藿香正气散。

【针刺取穴】中脘、天枢、气海、足三里、丰隆、太溪、照海、三阴交。

9. The Dark Red Tongue with White and Sticky, Thick Fur(Figure 9.9)

【Manifestations】 The tongue is reddened. The coating is white and sticky.

【Indications】 It is attributable to dampness pathogen complicated with Yin deficiency. In other words, this kind of tongues is formed in the case of Yin deficiency with internal fire, further suffering from over intake of rich food or cold food, which causes dampness retention. The constitutional Yin deficiency can lead to a red tongue. Dampness turbidity obstructs Yang Qi that can produce the sticky and white coating.

【Treatment】 It should be treated as dispersing dampness

and harmonizing the stomach. Huo-Xiang-Zheng-Qi-San(藿香正气散) is a proper medicine.

【Selection of acupoints】Zhongwan(Ren12), Tianshu(St25), Qihai(Ren6), Zusanli(St36), Fenglong(St40), Taixi(K3), Zhaohai(K6), Sanyinjiao(Sp6).

10. 红点舌白腻苔(图 9.10)

【舌象】舌的尖部红赤,并有红点,苔薄白腻。

【主病】心火亢盛。舌诊受脉诊影响很深,例如根据脉诊"上以候上,中以候中,下以候下"的原则,中医舌诊也将舌体做了脏腑分区,即舌尖部属心肺,舌中部属脾胃,舌根部属肝肾,舌边部属肝胆。本舌的尖部很红,故属心的火热证;红点也是热邪较盛的表现。

【治疗】清泻心火。方用导赤散或用朱砂安神丸。

【针刺取穴】少冲、神门、内关、曲泽、大椎、膻中。

10. The Red Dotted Tongue with Sticky and White Fur (Figure 9.10)

【Manifestations】The tongue tip is fresh red with some red spots. The coating is thin, sticky and white.

【Indications】It typifies hyperactivity of the heart fire. According to TCM, the principal of the tongue inspection is the same as that of the pulse, in detail, the up part detecting the up body, middle part showing the middle of body, and lower part reflecting the lower body. In the same way, the tongue tip corresponds to the heart and lung, while the center of the tongue to the spleen and stomach. The root of the tongue is related to the liver and kidney, and the sides to the liver and gallbladder. The picture as above shows obvious red at the tip, accordingly it indicates the heart fire syndrome. Those red spots are also the sign of excessive heat.

【Treatment】The treatment should be clearing away the heart fire. Dao-Chi-San(导赤散) or Zhu-Sha-An-Shen-Wan(朱砂安神丸) can be tried.

【Selection of acupoints】Shaochong(H9), Shenmen(H7), Neiguan(P6), Quze(P3), Dazhui(Du14), Shanzhong(Ren17).

第10章　绛　舌

1. 红绛裂纹无苔舌(图10.1)

【舌象】舌绛中有裂纹,无苔少津。

【主病】热盛伤阴,阴亏火旺。舌绛在外感病为热邪入血,在内伤为火旺,裂纹与无苔是热极伤阴。外感病为感染发热性病后期,如大叶性肺炎、乙型脑炎等,内伤病多见于心、脑血管病康复期。

【治疗】法当滋阴降火,凉血熄风,方用大定风珠加减。

【针刺取穴】大椎、曲泽、中冲、劳宫、列缺、照海、太溪、太冲。

Chapter 10　The Crimson Tongue

1. The Crimson Tongue with Fissures and no Fur(Figure 10.1)

【Manifestations】The tongue is crimson in color, showing dry and some fissures. It has no coating.

【Indications】It suggests that excessive heat has consumed Yin, leading to Yin deficiency and hyperactive fire. In the exogenous disease, the crimson tongue means invasion of the blood system by heat pathogen, While in the internal injury disease, it indicates excessive fire. The tongue body being fissured without coating reflects that heat pathogen is extremely excessive and Yin fluid has been injured. It is often seen in advanced period of infectious febrile diseases, such as lobar pneumonia, encephalitis B, or in the recovery period of cardiac cerebral vascular disease.

【Treatment】It should be treated as nourishing Yin and subduing fire, as well as cooling blood and stopping wind. Modified Da-Ding-Feng-Zhu(大定风珠) can be used.

【Selection of acupoints】Dazhui (Du14), Quze (P3), Zhongchong (P9), Laogong (P8), Lieque (Lu7), Zhaohai (K6), Taixi(K3), Taichong(Liv3).

2. **舌疮**(10.2)

【舌象】舌下肿痛，溃疡上覆白膜，舌下络脉青紫怒张，有出血点，舌绛娇嫩。

【主病】心经热毒，肝热舌血。舌疮以上焦心经郁火化毒为多，肝热则舌下出血。舌绛为热毒炽盛，热盛伤阴，气血瘀滞，故舌娇嫩而舌脉青紫怒张。舌疮多见于溃疡性舌炎、口腔炎，往往出现于急性热病后期。

【治序】法当清心败毒，泻肝解郁。方用泻心汤合龙胆泻肝汤。

【针刺取穴】大椎、少冲、中冲、曲泽、委中、太冲、足临泣。

2. The Ulcer of Tongue(Figure 10.2)

【Manifestations】The tongue shows an abscess beneath it. The ulcer surface grows a layer of membrane. The blood vessels under the tongue become enlarged and blue purplish with some bleeding dots. The tongue proper is tender.

【Indications】It is the syndrome of toxic heat in the heart meridian as well as the bleeding tongue due to the liver heat. For the ulcer of tongue is usually caused by heat toxin transformed from stagnant fire in the up-jiao and the heart meridian, and bleeding tongue by the liver heat. The crimson color indicates the excessive toxic heat, which can consume Yin fluid and lead to Qi-blood stagnancy, bringing the tongue tender in proper and blue vessels enlarged. Clinically, this kind of tongues can be seen in the cases of sore glossitis and stomatitis, which usually occurs in the late period of acute febrile diseases.

【Treatment】It should be treated as clearing the heart and removing toxin, as well as dispersing the liver and relieving depression. Xie-Xin-Tang (泻心汤) with Long-Dan-Xie-Gan-Tang(龙胆泻肝汤) can be adopted.

【Selection of acupoints】Dazhui(Du4), Shaochong(H9), Zhongchong(P9), Quze (P3), Weizhong (UB40), Taichong

(Liv3), Zulinqi(GB41).

3. 红绛舌中剥苔(图10.3)

【舌象】舌质红绛,苔薄白中剥,称“鸡心舌”,因其舌中无苔,形成椭圆形状,犹如鸡的心脏一样,故称“鸡心舌”。

【主病】胃热盛阴伤。这种舌象常见久病胃之气阴两虚,又遇饮食不节,或过食辛燥之品所致。舌质红绛为胃阴大伤之重症,苔薄白略腻为食滞胃肠,舌中部苔剥落为胃之气阴耗伤之象。临床常见于慢性胃炎、胰腺炎、肾盂肾炎、肺心病等慢性疾病的急性发作以及过敏性疾病、免疫系统的疾病,如风湿热或病毒性感染。

【治疗】清热生津、滋养胃阴。方用沙参麦冬汤。

【针刺取穴】脾俞、胃俞、肾俞、足三里、三阴交、太溪、曲池、合谷。

3. The Crimson Tongue with Exfoliated Fur in the Middle (Figure 10.3)

【Manifestations】 The tongue is crimson. The coating is thin, white and partly peeled in the center of the tongue. The peeled part is oval in shape seeming as the heart of a chicken, being termed “Chicken Heart Tongue”.

【Indications】It indicates Yin deficiency due to excessive heat of the stomach. Since this kind of tongues is usually seen in the case of prolonged disease that causes both Qi and Yin of stomach deficiency, again complicated with improper diet or overeating hot and spicy food. So the crimson tongue is a sign of severe damage of the stomach Yin, while the thin, white and sticky coating is the manifestation of stagnant food in the gastrointestinal tract. The exfoliated coating is a result of consumption of both Qi and Yin in the stomach. It is often seen on acute onset of diseases, such as chronic gastritis, pancreatitis, pyelonephritis, and pulmonary heart disease; or allergic diseases, immune system diseases, such as rheumatic fever, virus infections, etc.

【Treatment】 The treatment should be to clear away heat and produce body fluid, as well as to nourish the stomach Yin.

Sha-Shen-Mai-Dong-Tang(沙参麦冬汤) can be used.

【Selection of acupoints】Pishu(UB20), Weishu(UB21), Shenshu(UB23), Zusanli(St36), Sanyinjiao(Sp6), Taixi(K3), Quchi(LI11), Hegu(LI4).

4. 红绛芒刺舌,薄白少苔(图 10.4)

【舌象】舌质红绛,边尖部略显芒刺,舌苔薄白而稀少。

【主病】卫营合邪。舌质红绛而有芒刺是风热邪气内窜,深入营分之兆,是营分证候;苔薄白是风热外袭,肺卫失宣之象,属卫分证候,但已有伤阴之势;这种舌象见于卫营合邪证候。此证多见于现代医学麻疹,中医辨证属卫营合邪。

【治疗】两解卫营。方用银翘散加减。

【针刺取穴】少商、列缺、大椎、风池、风府、中冲、内关、血海、三阴交、膈俞。

4. The Red Tongue with Prickles and Less Thin and White Fur(Figure 10.4)

【Manifestations】The tongue is crimson, showing some red thorns at the edges and tip. The coating is thin, white and less.

【Indications】It indicates a combination of pathogens in the Ying-system and Wei-System. For the crimson tongue with red prickles is a sign of invasion of the Ying-system by wind heat from the exterior, it is the syndrome of Ying-system. The thin, white coating is the manifestation of the lung-Wei system failure in dispersion as a result of attack by exogenous wind heat. It indicates the syndrome of Wei-system as well as the tendency of Yin fluid impaired. So the tongue picture can be seen within the syndrome of combination of pathogens in both Ying and Wei systems, which occurs usually in the case of measles.

【Treatment】It should be treated as relieving the syndrome of both Wei and Ying systems. Modified Yin-Qiao-San(银翘散) can be used.

【Selection of acupoints】Shaoshang(Lu11), Lieque(Lu7), Dazhui(Du14), Fengchi(GB20), Fengfu(Du16),

Zhongchong(P9), Neiguan(P6), Xuehai(Sp10), Sanyinjiao(Sp6), Geshu(UB17).

5. 绛瘦舌,白腻花剥苔(图 10.5)

【舌象】舌深红为绛,略显瘦长;全舌白腻苔已部分剥落,称花剥苔。

【主病】在外感病为热入营血,热盛伤阴,湿浊未尽。在内伤病为肝肾阴液大伤,湿浊不化,胃气大伤。舌红绛瘦长,提示热邪深入营血,正气大伤;白腻苔部分剥落,说明湿浊未尽,胃气已伤;二者都是伤阴之象。

【治疗】清营凉血,滋阴活血。方用清营汤合犀角地黄汤加减。

【针刺取穴】膈俞、血海、三阴交、中冲、内关、公孙、太溪、足三里、丰隆。

5. The Crimson and Emaciated Tongue with White Sticky and Exfoliated Fur(Figure 10.5)

【Manifestations】The tongue being dark red belongs to the crimson tongue. It shows slightly thin and long. The white sticky coating has been partly peeled, so it is named an exfoliated tongue.

【Indications】If it appears in the exogenous disease, it denotes the invasion of Ying-blood system by pathogenic heat, and consumption of Yin fluid, as well as dampness turbidity existence. If it occurs in the internal injury disease, it indicates exhaustion of the liver and kidney Yin, retention of dampness turbidity, and heavy impairment of the stomach Qi. The crimson, thin and long tongue suggests that pathogenic heat has deeply invaded the Ying-Blood system and the vital Qi has been severely damaged. The white and sticky coating shows partly peeled, meaning turbid dampness still existing and the stomach Qi injured already. Both the tongue and coating present the sign of consumption of Yin.

【Treatment】When occurring in the infectious febrile disease (i.e. the exogenous disease), it should be treated as clearing the Ying-system and cooling the blood, in combination with nourishing Yin fluid and promoting blood circulation. Modified Qing-Ying-Tang（清营汤） with Xi-Jiao-Di-Huang-Tang（犀角地黄汤）can be used.

【Selection of acupoints】Geshu（UB17），Xuehai（Sp10），Sanyinjiao（Sp6），Zhongchong（P9），Neiguan（P6），Gongsun（Sp4），Taixi（K3），Zusanli（St36），Fenglong（St40）.

6. 红瘦舌，白腻花剥苔（图 10.6）

【舌象】舌质红而略瘦，苔白腻花剥。

【主病】阴虚内热，水湿停滞。多见久病脾胃气阴两虚，而有水湿内停之人。舌红略瘦，为胃阴大伤，虚热极盛；苔白腻，为脾胃气虚，水湿内停；花剥苔为虚火炽盛，阴液大伤，而湿邪未尽之象。大便不调，脉细数。临床多见于胃炎、肠炎及肝炎、胰腺炎等慢性炎症的急性发作的病变，或肝硬化、慢性肾炎、肾功能衰竭等疾病。

【治疗】滋补脾胃气阴，兼化湿浊。方用益胃汤加减。

【针刺取穴】中脘、天枢、气海、足三里、丰隆、阴陵泉、合谷、曲池、大椎。

6. The Red and Thin Tongue with White, Sticky and Exfoliated Fur（Figure 10.6）

【Manifestations】The tongue is red and slightly thin. The coating is white, sticky and partly peeled off.

【Indications】It is due to Yin deficiency and internal heat, as well as water dampness retention. It is usually seen in the case of prolonged diseases with deficiency of both Qi and Yin in the spleen and stomach, as well as water dampness retention. From the red and thin tongue, it can be known that the stomach Yin is heavily injured and deficient heat is extremely intense. From the white and sticky coating it is learnt that the spleen and stomach are insufficient so as to cause water dampness retention. The exfoliated coating is a sign of exhaustion of Yin fluid by intensely deficient fire, but dampness pathogen still existing. The symptoms linked with the tongue may be disorder of stool, thready and rapid pulse. In clinic, this kind of tongue can be seen at acute attack of some chronic inflammation diseases such as gastritis, enteritis, hepatitis, and pancreatitis, as well as the liver sclerosis, chronic nephritis, and renal failure, etc.

【Treatment】The method should be replenishing Qi and Yin of the spleen and stomach, as well as resolving turbid dampness. Modified Yi-Wei-Tang(益胃汤) can be tried.

【Selection of acupoints】Zhongwan(Ren12), Tianshu (St25), Qihai(Ren6), Zusanli(St36), Fenglong(St40), Yinlingquan(Sp9), Hegu(LI4), Quchi(LI11), Dazhui(Du14).

7. 红绛舌,白腻花剥苔(图 10.7)

【舌象】舌质红略绛,苔白腻花剥。

【主病】里热炽盛阴伤,水湿内停。这种舌象多见于久病之人,脾胃气阴两虚,又脾失健运,水湿内生,停聚体内。舌质深红而绛为里热炽盛,苔白腻为水湿内停,舌苔花剥又为腻苔,属脾胃气阴两伤而湿邪仍存之象。黄赤量少,脉濡数。临床可见慢性胃炎、肝胆病、肠炎、冠心病、高血压、肺心病、肾盂肾炎等病变的急性发作,属病情较重阶段。

【治疗】清热养阴,兼化湿浊。方用甘露消毒丹加减。

【针刺取穴】大椎、曲泽、中冲、足三里、丰隆、内庭、阴陵泉、三阴交、太溪。

7. The Crimson Tongue with White, Sticky and Exfoliated Fur(Figure 10.7)

【Manifestations】The tongue is red and light crimson. The coating is white, sticky and partly peeled off.

【Indications】It results from Yin consumption by excessive internal heat, as well as water dampness retention. For this type of tongues is often present in prolonged diseases marked by the deficiency of both Qi and Yin of the spleen and stomach, as well as the dysfunction of spleen in transforming, resulting in water dampness retention. The crimson tongue means excess of the internal heat, while the white coating shows retention of water dampness. The exfoliated coating is complicated with sticky coating, suggesting impairment of both Qi and Yin in the spleen and stomach and dampness retention. Some symptoms associated with the tongue may be scanty and dark urine, soft and rapid pulse. In clinic, the tongue may occurs at an acute stage of diseases, such as chronic gastritis, liver and gallbladder diseases, enteritis, coronary cardiac diseases, hypertension, pulmonary cardiac diseases, pyelonephritis, etc., belonging to the severe condition.

【Treatment】 It should be treated as clearing away heat and nourishing Yin, as well as resolving damp turbidity. Modified Gan-Lu-Xiao-Du-Dan(甘露消毒丹) can be used.

【Selection of acupoints】 Dazhui (Du14), Quze (P3), Zhongchong(P9), Zusanli (St36), Fenglong (St40), Neiting (St44), Yinlingquan(Sp9), Sanyinjiao(Sp6), Taixi(K3).

8. 红绛红点舌，薄白腻滑苔(图 10.8)

【舌象】舌质红绛而略显肿胀,夹有红点。苔薄白腻滑。

【主病】里热炽盛,湿浊内停之证。这种舌象多见急性热病,因所感受的火热邪气深重,热邪充斥人体,以致脏腑热盛之极,热入营血。舌红绛肿胀夹红点,为火热炽盛之象。苔薄白腻滑,是因秽浊湿邪因化热过快,而未能及时变为黄色所致。或脘腹胀满,尿黄,大便干燥,脉滑数。可见多种急性热病、手术后的炎症反应或中毒症,如各种传染性疾病、药物过敏、风湿热发作期、剥脱性皮炎或各种急性感染性疾病的炎症较重期间。

【治疗】清热解毒凉血。方用清瘟败毒饮加减(生石膏 30g、生连 9g、大青叶 15g、甘草 15g)。成药用牛黄安宫丸、牛黄清心丸、紫雪散。

【针刺取穴】足三里、上巨虚、内庭、中脘、天枢、中冲、内关、曲泽、大椎。

8. The Crimson Tongue with Red Dots, Covered by Thin, White, Sticky and Watery Fur(Figure 10.8)

【Manifestations】 The tongue is crimson and lightly swollen, showing some red spots. The coating is thin, white, sticky and watery.

【Indications】 It indicates excessive internal heat as well as dampness retention. Usually this type of tongues occurs in acute diseases. Since pathogenic fire-heat affected by the body is deeply serious, it dominates the whole body and makes the viscera as well as the Yin-blood system involved, which is learnt through the crimson and tongue with red spots. The thin, white and watery coating is attributable to turbid dampness. It transforms into heat too fast to bring the tongue into yellow. The symptoms linked with the tongue may be distending pain over epigastrium and abdomen, yellow urine, dry stool, slippery and rapid pulse, and so on. The tongue as above is able to appear in many acute febrile diseases, inflammatory reaction after operation, poisoning syndrome, various infectious diseases, drug allergy, rheumatic fever, exfoliative dermatitis, or in serious inflammation period of different acute infective diseases.

【Treatment】 The treatment should be to clear away heat and toxin, and to cool blood. Modified Qing-Wen-Bai-Du-Yin (清瘟败毒饮) can be used. For proprietary medicines, Niu-Huang-An-Gong-Wan(牛黄安宫丸), Niu-Huang-Qing-Xin-Wan(牛黄清心丸), and Zi-Xue-San(紫雪散) are suitable.

【Selection of acupoints】 Zusanli (St36), Shangjuxu (St37), Neiting(St44), Zhongwan(Ren12), Tianshu(St25), Zhongchong(P9), Neiguan(P6), Quze(P3), Dazhui(Du14).

9. 红绛舌，白腻淡黄苔(图 10.9)

【舌象】舌质红绛鲜泽,以舌边部为重,有突出舌面的红点。舌苔白腻淡黄。

【主病】肝火上炎。肝的阳气偏亢,故舌质色红绛鲜泽,舌边部为肝的分属部位,所以舌边尤其红赤。舌苔黄腻,也为肝经火热夹痰的征象。

【治疗】清肝泻火。方用龙胆泻肝汤。

【针刺取穴】大椎、太冲、足临泣、肝俞、胆俞、足三里、丰隆、内庭。

9. The Crimson Tongue with Sticky, White and Light Yellow Fur(Figure 10.9)

【Manifestation】 The tongue is fresh crimson, special at the edges and tip, with some red spots on the surface of the tongue. The coating is sticky, white, and light yellow.

【Indications】It is caused by hyperactivity of liver fire. Since the liver Yang is hyperactivity, it leads the tongue in fresh crimson color, especially on the sides and at the tip, because those parts are corresponding to the liver. The coating being yellow and sticky is also the sign of fire-heat within the liver meridian mixed with phlegm pathogen.

【Treatment】It should be treated as clearing the liver and eliminating fire. Long-Dan-Xie-Gan-Tang(龙胆泻肝汤) can be chosen.

【Selection of acupoints】Dazhui(Du14), Taichong(Liv3), Zulinqi(GB41), Ganshu(UB18), Danshu(UB19), Zusanli(St36), Fenglong(St40), Neiting(St44).

10. 红绛肿胀舌,根黄腐苔(图 10.10)

【舌象】舌质红绛而肿胀,舌中有裂纹而偏歪,苔根黄腐,舌尖无苔。

【主病】痰热内盛,气阴大伤。多因素体阴虚阳亢而痰湿内停,又阳亢化风,火热炽盛,阴液大伤所致。舌质红绛而肿胀,舌尖尤甚为心火炽盛,舌中有裂纹为阴液亏耗,舌偏歪为阳亢化风,舌根黄腐苔为痰热停滞之象。临床可见中风后遗症、冠心病、心肌梗死、癌症晚期等慢性消耗性病变或其它急性感染性疾病。

【治疗】清热滋阴,化痰熄风。方用镇肝熄风汤加减。

【针刺取穴】列缺、照海、中脘、天枢、气海、太冲、太溪、大椎、风池。

10. The Crimson and Swollen Tongue Covered by the Yellow and Curdy Fur at the Root(Figure 10.10)

【Manifestations】This is an enlarged and crimson tongue, with its body deviated and marked by some fissures on the surface. There is no coating at the tip, but some yellow and sticky coating seen at the root.

【Indications】This is attributed to excessive phlegm heat accompanied by Qi and Yin injured. In detail, the body has general Yin deficiency and Yang hyperactivity, as well as phlegm dampness retention. Hyperactive Yang transforms into wind, it results in fire-heat excess that consumes Yin fluid severely. From the crimson and swollen tongue, especially from the red tip we learn the excess of heart fire. From the fissured appearance we know consumption of Yin fluid. The deviated tongue is a sign of wind transformed from hyperactive Yang. The yellow and sticky coating at the root suggests phlegm heat stagnancy. In clinic, the tongue can be seen in diseases of wind-stroke sequela, coronary heart disease, myocardial infarction, advanced stage of cancer, chronic consumed diseases, or some other acute infective diseases.

【Treatment】 It should be treated as clearing away heat and nourishing Yin, as well as resolving phlegm and stopping wind. Modified Zhen-Gan-Xi-Feng-Tang(镇肝熄风汤) is suitable.

【Selection of acupoints】 Lieque(Lu7), Zhaohai(K6), Zhongwan(Ren12), Tianshu(St25), Qihai(Ren6), Taichong(Liv3), Taixi(K3), Dazhui(Du14), Fengchi(GB20).

第11章 青紫舌

1. **暗紫黑点舌,薄白透明苔**(图 11.1)

【舌象】舌暗紫胖嫩,略显齿痕,边尖散布无数红黑点。舌面被覆着极薄的一层透明苔,好像浮胖,似苔非苔,尖部明亮小点是津液反光。

【主病】血蕴湿热,营热挟瘀,水湿上犯。湿热邪盛,瘟毒入血,热毒乘心,故边尖见大量红黑星点。湿热郁滞,气滞血瘀,故舌质紫暗。湿热困脾,脾虚则湿滞不化,故舌胖嫩而有齿痕。水湿之邪上泛,故见薄白透明苔。

【治疗】用凉血活血,益气化湿法。方用清营汤加减。

【针刺取穴】心俞、膈俞、血海、三阴交、足三里、阴陵泉。

Chapter 11 The Blue and Purple Tongue

1. The Dark Purple Tongue with Black Dots Covered by the Thin, White and Clarity Coating(Figure 11.1)

【Manifestations】This tongue shows dark purple color. Its body is enlarged, teeth printed and tender, appearing many reddened or black dots at the edges and tip. The surface is covered by a layer of extremely thin and clarity coating as if puffy and no coating. The bright dots at the tip are actually light reflection by liquid.

【Indications】It is attributable to dampness heat accumulated in the Ying and blood system, the heat pathogen of Ying system combined with blood stasis, water dampness pathogen floating upwards. Since dampness heat is so excessive that it can transform into toxin and then invade the blood system, the heart involved, bringing about many red or black dots at the tip and edges. Furthermore, Dampness heat accumulation can cause blood stagnant, which is shown by the dark purple color of tongue. In another hand, damp-heat pathogen blocks the spleen function of transportation, dampness stagnancy failing to be resolved, thus the tongue is enlarged and printed by teeth. The thin and clarify coating is formed as a result of water dampness floating upwards.

【Treatment】It should be treated as cooling blood and promoting blood circulation, as well as benefiting Qi and resolving dampness. Modified Qing-Ying-Tang(清营汤) can be used.

【Selection of acupoints】Xinshu(UB15), Geshu(UB17), Xuehai(Sp10), Sanyinjiao(Sp6), Zusanli(St36), Yinlingquan (Sp9).

2. 淡紫瘀点舌,透明苔(图 11.2)

【舌象】舌质淡紫,夹瘀点,舌体偏胖,苔白透明。

【主病】阳虚水停,血虚瘀血。多因素体阳虚,无力推动血液和水液运行,致血行瘀滞,水液代谢失调,而瘀血水湿内停。舌体偏胖,舌质淡为阳气虚弱,舌淡暗夹瘀点为血虚血瘀之象,苔白透明为水湿之邪停滞所致。大便不调,或咳喘痰多,或尿少,小便不利,水肿,脉虚或结代。临床见于慢性肾病、肾功能衰竭、心力衰竭、各种血液病、癌症晚期或各种慢性消耗性疾病。

【治疗】温阳化湿,养血活血。方用苓桂术甘汤加味。

【针刺取穴】关元、气海、足三里、阴陵泉、三阴交、脾俞、肾俞。

2. The Light Purple Tongue with Dark Spots Covered by Clarity Coating(Figure 11.2)

【Manifestations】This is a purplish tongue with some petechia. Its body is puffy, and the coating is clarity.

【Indications】It suggests Yang deficiency, water retention, as well as blood deficiency and stasis. Since Yang is insufficient, it fails to promote blood circulation and water metabolism, leading to blood stagnation and water dampness retention. From the puffy and pale tongue we can know Yang deficient. From its dark light color and petechia we may learn blood deficiency and stagnation. The white and clarity coating is due to dampness retention. Some symptoms may be seen as loose stool, or coughing profuse sputum, or scanty urine, dysuria, swollen, weak pulse or intermitted pulse. This type of tongue can occur in chronic nephropathy, renal failure, heart failure, and hematopathy, cancer in advanced stage, or some chronic consumption diseases, etc.

【Treatment】The treatment should be warming Yang and resolving dampness, as well as nourishing blood and promoting blood circulation. Modified Ling-Gui-Zhu-Gan-Tang(苓桂术甘汤) is suitable.

【Selection of acupoints】Guanyuan (Ren4), Qihai (Ren6), Zusanli (St36), Yinlingquan (Sp9), Sanyinjiao (Sp6), Pishu(UB20), Shenshu(UB23).

3. 淡紫胖嫩舌,薄白润苔(图 11.3)

【舌象】舌淡紫胖嫩,边尖隐约可见小黑点,中有裂纹;苔薄白而润,右侧根部尚残留黄厚腻苔,左边也残留少许白腻苔。

【主病】湿热蕴于血分,气血阻滞,经治疗黄厚腻苔逐渐化退,胃气渐复,新生薄白苔,但余邪未清,脾胃已伤。胖嫩属气虚,纵裂为中焦不足,淡紫与黑点说明血分尚有瘀滞,舌根黄腻苔为下焦湿热尚未全部清除。可见于传染性肝炎恢复期、迁延性肝炎、慢性肝炎、肠伤寒康复期、痢疾康复期等。

【治疗】用健脾化湿,理气活血法。方用六君子汤合逍遥散加减。

【针刺取穴】肝俞、胆俞、脾俞、足三里、阴陵泉、三阴交。

3. The Purplish, Enlarged and Tender Tongue Covered by Thin Whiteness and Moist Coating(Figure 11.3)

【Manifestations】This tongue shows purplish, puffy and tender, with some black dots vaguely seen on the sides and tip. The tongue is fissured, covered by the thin whiteness and moist coating. It appears yellow thickness and greasy coating on the right root part and some white and greasy coating on the left part.

【Indications】 It means that dampness heat accumulates within blood and results in blood stasis. After treatment, the yellow thickness and greasy coating disappears gradually, meanwhile the stomach Qi is recovered, the thin and white coating newly produced, but some pathogen still rested and the spleen and stomach already injured. The puffy and tender of tongue pertains to Qi deficiency. Fissured tongue is due to the middle jiao insufficient. Purplish color and black dots suggest blood stasis. The yellow and greasy coating in the root tongue indicates dampness heat of the lower-Jiao without eliminated. The tongue picture can be seen in recovery period of infectious hepatitis, persistent hepatitis, chronic hepatitis, or ileotyphus, or dysentery, etc.

【Treatment】 The treatment should be invigorating the spleen and eliminating dampness, as well as promoting Qi and blood circulation. Modified Liu-Jun-Zi-Tang(六君子汤) combined with Xiao-Yao-San(逍遥散) can be used.

【Selection of acupoints】 Ganshu (UB18), Danshu (UB19), Pishu(UB20), Zusanli(St36), Yinlingquan(Sp9), Sanyinjiao(Sp6).

4. 暗紫红点舌,白腻干苔(图 11.4)

【舌象】舌质紫暗,舌尖略红,有明显红点;舌苔白腻而干,中部厚而淡黄。

【主病】痰热湿浊瘀阻血分。湿浊、痰饮蕴久化热,故见舌尖红点,苔腻淡黄,干燥无津。痰浊阻滞,血脉不畅,故舌紫暗。临床可见胸闷纳呆,呕恶,心胸闷痛或压榨样疼痛,痛有定处,或如刺如绞向肩背放射;痰多粘稠,便秘尿黄等,属痰热湿浊瘀阻的症状。

【治疗】法当化痰清热,理气活血。方用黄连温胆汤加减。

【针刺取穴】中脘、天枢、气海、足三里、上巨虚、内庭、内关、公孙。

4. The Dark Purple Tongue with Some Red Dots Covered by White, Greasy and Dry Coating(Figure 11.4)

【Manifestations】This is a dim purple tongue, but the tip is slightly red and shows some red spots. The coating is white, greasy and dryness, with its middle thickness and light yellow.

【Indications】The reason for the tongue is obstruction of blood by phlegm heat and damp turbidity. For turbid dampness and phlegm fluid may transform into heat after long period stagnation, they can manifest as red spots, light yellow and greasy coating with dryness. Phlegm turbidity blocks blood circulation, leading to unsmooth flow of blood, which gives rise to darkness of the tongue. In clinic, fullness of the chest, poor digestion, nausea and vomiting, distending pain or depressing pain over heart region and chest, the pain characterized by fixation or radiation to the back, profuse and thickness sputum, constipation, and yellow urine, can be seen. They belong to symptoms of phlegm heat and turbid dampness obstructing blood circulation.

【Treatment】The treatment method should be eliminating phlegm heat and promoting circulation of Qi and blood. Modified Huang-Lian-Wen-Dan-Tang(黄连温胆汤) can be chosen.

【Selection of acupoints】Zhongwan (Ren12), Tianshu (St25), Qihai (Ren6), Zusánli (St36), Shangjuxu (St37), Neiting(St44), Neiguan(P6), Gongsun(Sp4).

5. 暗紫偏歪舌，白腻湿润苔(图 11.5)

【舌象】舌暗紫略胖歪斜，尖部隐隐可见红点，舌苔白腻湿润，满布舌上。

【主病】湿浊内蕴，风痰阻络。舌胖与满舌白腻湿润苔，说明湿浊内蕴；湿郁成痰，风邪挟痰走窜经络，气血瘀阻，故舌见歪斜，色紫暗滞，风痰化火，则舌尖见红点。此舌常见于脑血栓形成等脑血管病。

【治疗】法当祛风化痰、活血通络。方用牵正散加味。

【针刺取穴】中脘、天枢、气海、足三里、丰隆、阳陵泉、后溪、申脉。

5. The Dark Purple and Deviated Tongue Covered by White, Greasy and Moist Coating(Figure 11.5)

【Manifestations】 The tongue is dim purple color and slightly enlarged, turning to one side. On its tip there are some red dots vaguely seen. The coating is white, greasy and moisture, fully distributed on the whole tongue.

【Indications】 The reason is turbid dampness retention as well as collateral obstruction by wind phlegm. The enlarged tongue with greasy whiteness and moist coating suggests turbid dampness retention. Stagnant dampness may change into phlegm that can be taken by the internal wind and moved along the meridians, leading to obstruction of Qi and blood, leaving the tongue turned to one side and marked with purple darkness color. The red spots on the tip are the sign of fire transformed from wind phlegm. This type of tongue often occurs in cerebral vascular diseases such as thrombosis.

【Treatment】 The method is to expel wind and resolve phlegm, as well as promote blood circulation and dredge the collateral. Modified Qian-Zheng-San(牵正散) can be chosen.

【Selection of acupoints】 Zhongwan (Ren12), Tianshu (St25), Qihai(Ren6), Zusanli(St36), Fenglong(St40), Yanglingquan(GB34), Houxi(SI3), Shenmai(UB62).

6. 淡紫舌，薄白腻苔(图 11.6)

【舌象】舌质淡红，略带暗紫，左边稍有齿痕；舌苔薄白而腻，根部略厚。

【主病】饮酒外感风寒，湿浊阻滞气血。舌淡红紫暗属于淡紫，可见于经常嗜酒者，由于酒毒日积月累，使舌色变紫。感受风寒邪气，初起病邪在表，舌苔多薄白。根部厚腻苔，主下焦内蕴湿邪，湿浊阻滞气血，可使舌色紫暗。

【治疗】感寒湿者可用解表散寒，芳香化浊法。方用藿香正气散加减。

【针刺取穴】风池、尺泽、列缺、大椎、足三里、丰隆、曲池、合谷。

6. The Purplish Tongue with White and Greasy Coating (Figure 11.6)

【Manifestations】 The tongue is light red and purplish, appearing some teeth prints on left side. The coating is thin whiteness and greasy, slight thickness seen on the root part.

【Indications】The cause for the tongue may be the alcoholism people attacked by wind cold pathogens, Qi and blood obstructed by damp turbidity. Usually the light red and purplish tongue is seen in sot, since accumulation of alcohol poison can lead the tongue into purple color. The exogenous wind cold invades the exterior of body initially, manifesting as the thin and white coating. Thick greasy coating on the root part of tongue means dampness pathogen stagnating in the lower-Jiao. It can obstruct Qi and blood circulation, resulting in the darkness purple tongue.

【Treatment】It can be treated as relieving the exterior syndrome and expelling coldness, combined with resolving dampness turbidity with fragrant medicine. Modified Huo-Xiang-Zheng-Qi-San(藿香正气散) is suitable.

【Selection of acupoints】Fengchi(GB20), Chize(Lu5), Lieque(Lu7), Dazhui(Du14), Zusanli(St36), Fenglong(St40), Quchi(LI11), Hegu(LI4).

7. 青紫淡嫩舌，薄白水滑苔(图 11.7)

【舌象】舌淡青紫胖嫩，略显齿痕，舌苔薄白水滑，根部稍见淡黄。

【主病】脾肾气虚，湿阻血瘀，虚火上浮。舌淡胖嫩主气虚，脾肾气虚，寒水不化，故苔薄白水滑。稍见淡黄为虚热之证，口周小疖(毛囊炎)是虚火所致。寒滞湿阻，血瘀故见舌青紫。可见于糖尿病后期合并的冠心病。

【治疗】法当温肾健脾，利湿活血，引火归元。方用补中益气汤合济生肾气丸加减。

【针刺取穴】脾俞、肾俞、命门、三阴交、阴陵泉、足三里、太冲。

7. The Bluish Purple and Tender Tongue with Thin Whiteness and Watery Coating(Figure 11.7)

【Manifestations】This is an enlarged and tender tongue showing bluish purple color and teeth prints. The coating is thin whiteness and watery, light yellow seen on the root part.

【Indications】 It suggests the spleen and kidney deficiency, dampness retention and blood stasis, as well as upward flaming of deficient fire. Generally, the pale, enlarged and tender tongue pertains to Qi deficiency. Because the spleen and kidney Qi is insufficient, it fails to distribute cold water, bringing about the watery, thin and white coating. The light yellow color on the root is the manifestation of deficient heat, while the rashes around mouth are due to flaming fire. On the other hand, cold dampness pathogen obstructs blood circulation and causes blood stasis, leading to the bluish purple tongue. It can occur in the late period of diabetes complicated with coronary heart disease.

【Treatment】 The suitable method is to warm the kidney and invigorate the spleen, to excrete dampness and promote blood circulation, as well as to conduct fire back to its origin. Modified Bu-Zhong-Yi-Qi-Tang(补中益气汤) with Ji-Shèng-Shen-Qi-Wan(济生肾气丸) can be used.

【Selection of acupoints】Pishu(UB20), Shenshu(UB23), Mingmen(Du4), Sanyinjiao(Sp6), Yinlingquan(Sp9), Zusanli (St36), Taichong(Liv3).

8. 淡紫红点舌,白腻淡黄苔(图 11.8)

【舌象】舌色淡紫,边尖隐约可见红点,舌苔白腻不厚,中部略显淡黄。

【主病】外感寒湿,有入里化热之势。舌淡紫苔白腻是外感寒湿之象,苔不厚为邪仍在表,边有红点,中部淡黄,说明有化热入血之势。胸闷咳喘,痰白稀薄、纳呆尿黄,头痛身重等。慢性支气管炎急性发作、上呼吸道感染、流行性感冒等病。

【治疗】法当散寒祛湿,兼清内热。方用藿香正气散加减。

【针刺取穴】风池、太渊、列缺、肺俞、脾俞、胃俞。

8. The Purplish Tongue with Red Spots Covered by Greasy, White and Yellowish Coating(Figure 11.8)

【Manifestations】 It is a pale purple tongue with some red dots vaguely seen on the sides and tip. Its coating is white, greasy and thin, showing light yellow on the center.

【Indications】It is due to exogenous dampness cold that tends to turn into heat. The pale purple tongue and greasy whiteness coating are the sign of exogenous cold dampness. It is thin meaning the pathogen still in the exterior. The red spots on the sides with light yellow coating in the middle suggest the heat tendency and invasion of the interior. The symptoms linked to the tongue may be stuffy chest, asthma and coughing, white and thin sputum, poor appetite, yellow urine, headache and heavy sensation of the body, and so on. It can be seen in acute onset of chronic bronchitis, up respiratory tract infection, flu, etc.

【Treatment】It should be treated as expelling cold dampness as well as clearing away internal heat. Modified Huo-Xiang-Zheng-Qi-San(藿香正气散) can be chosen.

【Selection of acupoints】Fengchi(GB20), Taiyuan(Lu9), Lieque (Lu7), Feishu (UB13), Pishu (UB20), Weishu (UB21).

9. 淡紫胖嫩舌,薄腻中灰苔(图 11.9)

【舌象】舌淡紫胖嫩,略显齿痕,尖有暗红小点。苔薄白腻似透明,中根部淡黄带灰。

【主病】气虚血瘀,湿郁化热。舌体胖嫩、齿痕、色淡皆气虚阳虚之象,阳虚气虚而血瘀,故舌色紫暗。脾虚湿留,故苔白腻透明。邪不甚则苔薄,湿郁久则化热,虚热上浮见舌苔淡黄而灰。见于慢性肾炎、冠心病、再生障碍性贫血。

【治疗】法当益气活血,温阳利湿清热。方用温脾汤合补阳还五汤。

【针刺取穴】中脘、天枢、气海、关元、血海、膈俞、三阴交、阴陵泉。

9. The Purplish and Enlarged Tongue Covered by Thin and Greasy Coating Showing Gray Fur in the Middle(Figure 11.9)

【Manifestations】The tongue is pale and purple in color, enlarged and tender in property, appearing teeth prints, some dark red and tiny spots seen on the tip. The coating being thin, greasy and white seems clarity, with yellowish and gray color present in the center and root region.

【Indications】The cause of it is Qi deficiency and blood stasis, as well as dampness retention turning into heat. The tongue body marked by puffy, tender, tooth-prints, and pale color means Yang deficiency. The insufficient Yang and Qi result in blood stasis, giving rise to the purple darkness tongue. The deficient spleen causes dampness retention, so the coating is white, greasy and clarity. The pathogen is not excess, thus the coating manifests thin. The dampness stagnating long period can change into heat, and deficient heat may flame upwards, leading to the yellowish and gray coating. It can be seen in chronic nephritis, coronary heart disease, and aplastic anemia, etc.

【Treatment】It should be treated as benefiting Qi and promoting blood circulation, as well as warming Yang, and eliminating dampness heat. Modified Wen-Pi-Tang(温脾汤) with Bu-Yang-Huan-Wu-Tang(补阳还五汤) can be tried.

【Selection of acupoints】Zhongwan(Ren12), Tianshu(St25), Qihai(Ren6), Guanyaun(Ren4), Xuehai(Sp10), Geshu(UB17), Sanyinjiao(Sp6), Yinlingquan(Sp9).

10. **绛紫舌,黄腻燥裂苔(图 11.10)**

【舌象】舌质绛紫苍老,舌苔由白转黄,中根部厚腻燥裂。

【主病】血热深重,胃肠实热。绛紫由红舌发展而来,说明邪热深入血分,或嗜酒者由酒毒蕴结,脏腑实热。中根部黄腻燥裂苔,是胃肠实热积滞,化燥伤津所致。可见于流行性乙型脑炎、出血热、流行性脑膜炎等,往往伴有热盛动风、热盛动血等,也可见于溃疡病穿孔、急性阑尾炎、肠伤寒、肠梗阻等急腹症。

【治疗】热入营血者,宜清营凉血。方用清营汤合犀角地黄汤加减。胃肠实热者,宜通腹泄热,方用大承气汤。

【针刺取穴】曲池、内庭、大椎、足三里、上巨虚、血海、太冲、膈俞。

10. The Crimson Purple Tongue with Yellow, Greasy and

Dryness Coating Showing Fissures(Figure 11.10)

【Manifestations】 This is a rough, crimson and purple tongue. The coating is changing from white color to yellow, in its middle and root region showing thick, greasy, dryness and fissures.

【Indications】 It indicates serious blood heat as well as excessive heat in the gastrointestinal tract. The crimson purple tongue is developed from red tongue, suggesting invasion of blood by pathogenic heat, or excessive heat in the viscera due to alcoholism. The yellow, greasy, dryness and fissured coating seen in the middle and root part results from consumption of body fluid by excessive heat stagnancy in the gastrointestinal tract. It can be seen in epidemic encephalitis B, hemorrhagic fever, and epidemic meningitis, which is often combined with the symptoms of wind or bleeding caused by excessive heat; as well as in ulcer disease with perforation, acute appendicitis, ileotyphus, ileus, and so on, which belong to acute abdomen.

【Treatment】 For invasion of Ying and blood system, the treatment should be clearing Ying and cooling blood. Modified Qing-Ying-Tang(清营汤) with Xi-Jiao-Di-Huang-Tang(犀角地黄汤) can be used. For excessive heat in the gastrointestinal tract, the method is to eliminate heat by purging the bowels. Da-Cheng-Qi-Tang(大承气汤) can be tried.

【Selection of acupoints】 Quchi(LI11), Neiting(St44), Dazhui(Du14), Zusanli(St36), Shangjuxu(St37), Xuhai(Sp37), Taichong(Liv3), Geshu(UB17).

方剂索引（Index of Formulae）

中文	拼 音	英 文	拉丁文
·八珍汤	Ba-Zhen-Tang Eight Precious Ingredients Decoction		
人参	Ren Shen	Ginseng	Radix Ginseng
白芍药	Bai Shao Yao	White peony root	Radix Paeoniae Alba
白术	Bai zhu	White atractylodes	Rhizoma Atractylodis Macrocephalae
川芎	Chuan Xiong	Ligusticum rhizome	Rhizoma Chuanxiong
茯苓	Fu Ling	Poria	Poria
熟地	Shu Di	Prepared rehmannia root	Radix Rehmanniae Praeparata
甘草	Gan Cao	Licorice root	Radix Glycyrrhizae
生姜	Sheng Jiang	Fresh ginger	Rhizoma Zingiberis Recens
当归	Dang Gui	Chinese angelica root	Radix Angelicae Sinensis
大枣	Da Zao	Jujube	Fructus Ziziphus Jujubae
·白虎加苍术汤	Bai-Hu-Jia-Cang-Zhu-Tang White Tiger decoction with Chinese Atractylodes		
生石膏	Sheng Shi Gao	Gypsum	Gypsum Fibrosum
知母	Zhi Mu	Anemarrhena rhizome	Rhizoma Anemarrhenae
甘草	Gan Cao	Licorice root	Radix Glycyrrhizae
粳米	Jing Mi	Rice	Semen Oryzae
苍术	Cang Zhu	Atractylodes rhizome	Rhizoma Atractylodis

·补中益气汤 Bu-Zhong-Yi-Qi-Tang

The Middle-Reinforcing and Qi-Benefiting Decoction

人参	Ren Shen	Ginseng	Radix Ginseng
黄芪	Huang Qi	Astragalus root	Radix Astragali
白术	Bai Zhu	White atractylodes	Rhizoma Atractylodis Macrocephalae
甘草	Gan Cao	Licorice root	Radix Glycyrrhizae
当归	Dang Gui	Chinese angelica root	Radix Angelicae Sinensis
陈皮	Chen Pi	Tangerine peel	Pericarpium Citri Reticulatae
升麻	Sheng Ma	Cimicifuga rhizome	Rhizoma Cimicifugae
柴胡	Chai Hu	Bupleurum root	Radix Bupleuri

·保和丸 Bao-He-Wan

Harmony-Preserving Pills

半夏	Ban Xia	Pinellia	Rhizoma Pinelliae
神曲	Shen Qu	Medicated leaven	Massa Fermentata Medicinalis
山楂	Shan Zha	Hawthorn fruit	Fructus Crataegi
茯苓	Fu Ling	Poria	Poria
陈皮	Chen Pi	Tangerine peel	Pericarpium Citri Reticulatae
连翘	Lian Qiao	Forsythia fruit	Fructus Forsythiae
莱菔子	Lai Fu Zi	Radish Seed	Semen Raphani

·柴胡疏肝饮 Chai-Hu-Shu-Gan-Yin

Bupleurum Liver-Soothing Decoction

柴胡	Chai Hu	Bupleurum root	Radix Bupleuri
枳壳	Zhi Qiao	Bitter orange	Fructus Aurantii
白芍药	Bai Shao Yao	White peony root	Radix Paeoniae Alba
甘草	Gan Cao	Licorice root	Radix Glycyrrhizae
香附	Xiang Fu	Cyperus tuber	Rhizoma Cyperi
川芎	Chuan Xiong	Ligusticum rhizome	Rhizoma Chuanxiong

·大定风珠 Da-Ding-Feng-Zhu
Great Wind-Stabilizing Decotion

白芍药	Bai Shao Yao	White peony root	Radix Paeoniae Alba
阿胶	E Jiao	Gelatin	Colla Corii Asini
生龟板	Sheng Gui Ban	Tortoise plastron	Plastrum Testudinis
生地黄	Sheng Di Huang	Rehmannia root	Radix Rehmanniae
火麻仁	Huo Ma Ren	Cannabis seed	Fructus Cannabis
五味子	Wu Wei Zi	Schisandra fruit	Fructus Schisandrae
生牡蛎	Sheng Mu Li	Oyster shell	Concha Ostreae
麦冬	Mai Dong	Ophiopogon root	Radiax Ophiopogonis
炙甘草	Zhi Gan Cao	Prepared licorice root	Radix Glycyrrhizae Preparata
鸡子黄	Ji Zi Huang	Yolk	Yolk
生鳖甲	Sheng Bie Jia	Tortoise shell	Carapax Trionycis

·当归补血汤 Dang-Gui-Bu-Xue-Tang
Chinese Angelica Dectioon for Replenishing Blood

当归	Dang Gui	Chinese angelica root	Radix Angelicae Sinensis
黄芪	Huang Qi	Astragalus root	Radix Astragali

·导赤散 Dao-Chi-San
Powder for Reducing Heart Fire

生地黄	Sheng Di Huang	Rehmannia root	Radix Rehmanniae
木通	Mu Tong	Akebia stem	Caulis Akebiae
竹叶	Zhu Ye	Bamboo shavings	Folium Bambusae
甘草	Gan Cao	Licorice root	Radix Glycyrrhizae

·二冬汤 Er-Dong-Tang

Two Dong Decotion

天冬	Tian Dong	Asparagus root	Radix Asparagi
麦冬	Mai Dong	Ophiopogon root	Radiax Ophiopogonis
天花粉	Tian Hua Fen	Trichosanthes root	Radix Trichosanthis
黄芩	Huang Qin	Scutellaria root	Radix Scutellariae
知母	Zhi Mu	Anemarrhena rhizome	Rhizoma Anemarrhenae
甘草	Gan Cao	Licorice root	Radix Glycyrrhizae
人参	Ren Shen	Ginseng	Radix Ginseng
荷叶	He Ye	Leaf of nelumbo nucifera	Folium Nelumbinis

·二妙丸 Er-Miao-Wan

Two Wonderful Herbs Powder

黄柏	Huang Bai	Phellodendron bark	Cortex Phellodendri
苍术	Cang Zhu	Atractylodes rhizome	Rhizoma Atractylodis

·附子理中汤 Fu-Zi-Li-Zhong-Tang

Aconite Middle-Regulating Decotion

附子	Fu Zi	Aconite	Radix Aconiti Praeparata
干姜	Gan Jiang	Dry ginger	Rhizoma Zingiberis
党参	Dang Sheng	Pilose asiabell root	Radix Angelicae Sinensis
白术	Bai Zhu	White atractylodes	Rhizoma Atractylodis Macrocephalae
甘草	Gan Cao	Licorice root	Radix Glycyrrhizae

·甘露消毒丹 Gan-Lu-Xiao-Du-Dan

Sweet Dew Detoxicatioon pellets

滑石	Hua Shi	Talc	Talcum
茵陈	Yin Chen	Evergreen artemisia	Herba Artemisiae Capillaris
黄芩	Huang Qin	Scutellaria root	Radix Scutellariae
石菖蒲	Shi Chang Pu	Acorus rhizome	Rhizoma Acori Graminei
川贝母	Chuan Bei Mu	Tendrilled Fritillary bulb	Bulbus Fritillariae Cirrhosae
藿香	Huo Xiang	Agastache	Herba Agastachis
射干	She Gan	Belamcanda rhizome	Rhizoma Belamcandae
连翘	Lian Qiao	Forsythia fruit	Fructus Forsythiae
薄荷	Bo He	Mentha	Herba Menthae
白蔻仁	Bai Kou Ren	Cluster	Semen Cardamomi Rotundi

·膈下逐瘀汤 Ge-Xia-Zhu-Yu-Tang

Decotion for Dissipating Blood Stasis Under Diaphragm

五灵脂	Wu Ling Zhi	Trogopterus dung	Faeces Trogopterorum
当归	Dang Gui	Chinese angelica root	Radix Angelicae Sinensis
川芎	Chuan Xiong	Ligusticum rhizome	Rhizoma Chuanxiong
桃仁	Tao Ren	Persica seed	Semen Persicae
丹皮	Dan Pi	Mutan bark	Cortex Moutan Radicis
赤芍药	Chi Shao Yao	Red peony	Radix Paeoniae Rubra
乌药	Wu Yao	Lindera root	Radix Linderae

延胡索	Yan Hu Suo	Corydalis tuber	Rhizoma Corydalis
甘草	Gan Cao	Licorice root	Radix Glycyrrhizae
香附	Xiang Fu	Cyperus tuber	Rhizoma Cyperi
红花	Hong Hua	Carthamus	Flos Carthami
枳壳	Zhi Qiao	Bitter orange	Fructus Aurantii

·归脾汤 Gui-Pi-Tang

Decotion for Invigorating the Spleen and Heart

黄芪	Huang Qi	Astragalus root	Radix Astragali
党参	Dang Sheng	Pilose asiabell root	Radix Angelicae Sinensis
白术	Bai Zhu	White atractylodes	Rhizoma Atractylodis Macrocephalae
茯神	Fu Shen	Poria	Poria
酸枣仁	Suan Zao Ren	Wild jujube	Semen Ziziphi Spinosae
龙眼肉	Long Yan Rou	Longan aril	Arillus Longan
木香	Mu Xiang	Saussurea root	Radix Saussureae
炙甘草	Zhi Gan Cao	Prepared licorice root	Radix Glycyrrhizae Preparata
当归	Dang Gui	Chinese angelica root	Radix Angelicae Sinensis
远志	Yuan Zhi	Polygala root	Radix Polygalae
生姜	Sheng Jiang	Fresh ginger	Rhizoma Zingiberis Recens
大枣	Da Zao	Jujube	Fructus Ziziphus Jujubae

·黄芩滑石汤 Huang-Qin-Hua-Shi-Tang

Scutellaria and Talc Decoction

黄芩	Huang Qin	Scutellaria root	Radix Scutellariae

滑石	Hua Shi	Talc	Talcum
茯苓皮	Fu Ling Pi	Poria	Poria
大腹皮	Da Fu Pi	Areca peel	Pericarpium Arecae
白蔻仁	Bai Kou Ren	Cluster	Semen Cardamomi Rotundi
通草	Tong Cao	Akebia stem	Caulis Akebiae
猪苓	Zhu Ling	Polyporus	Polyporus Umbellatus
藿香	Huo Xiang	Agastache	Herba Agastachis
佩兰	Pei Lan	Eupatorium	Herba Eupatorii

·黄连解毒汤 Huang-Lian-Jie-Du-Tang

Coptis Detoxicating Decoction

黄连	Huang Lian	Coptis root and rhizome	Rhizoma Coptidis
黄芩	Huang Qin	Scutellaria root	Radix Scutellariae
黄柏	Huang Bai	Phellodendron bark	Cortex Phellodendri
栀子	Zhi Zi	Gardenia fruit	Fructus Gardeniae

·黄连温胆汤 Huang-Lian-Wen-Dan-Tang

Coptis Decotion for Gallbladder Heat

黄连	Huang Lian	Coptis root and rhizome	Rhizoma Coptidis
半夏	Ban Xia	Pinellia	Rhizoma Pinelliae
陈皮	Chen Pi	Tangerine peel	Pericarpium Citri Reticulatae
茯苓	Fu Ling	Poria	Poria
甘草	Gan Cao	Licorice root	Radix Glycyrrhizae
枳实	Zhi Shi	Immature bitter orange	Fructus Aurantii Immaturus
竹茹	Zhu Ru	Bamboo shavings	Caulus Bambusae in Taenis

大枣	Da Zao	Jujube	Fructus Ziziphus Jujubae

·**藿香正气散** Huo-Xiang-Zheng-Qi-San

Powder of Agastache for Restoring Health

藿香	Huo Xiang	Agastache	Herba Agastachis
白芷	Bai Zhi	Angelica	Radix Angelicae Dahuricae
紫苏	Zi Su	Perilla leaf	Folium Perillae
桔梗	Jie Geng	Platycodon root	Radix Platycodi
白术	Bai Zhu	White atractylodes	Rhizoma Atractylodis Macrocephalae
厚朴	Hou Po	Magnolia bark	Cortex Magnoliae Officinalis
半夏曲	Ban Xia Qu	Pinellia	Rhizoma Pinelliae
大腹皮	Da Fu Pi	Areca peel	Pericarpium Arecae
茯苓	Fu Ling	Poria	Poria
橘皮	Ju Pi	Tangerine peel	Pericarpium Citri Rticulatae
甘草	Gan Cao	Licorice root	Radix Glycyrrhizae
大枣	Da Zao	Jujube	Fructus Ziziphus Jujubae

·**加味异功散** Jia-Wei-Yi-Gong-San

Modicied Marvelous Powder

党参	Dang Shen	Pilose asiabell root	Radix Angelicae Sinensis
白术	Bai Zhu	White atractylodes	Rhizoma Atractylodis Macrocephalae
白芍药	Bai Shao Yao	White peony root	Radix Paeoniae Alba
橘红	Ju Hong	Pilose asiabell root	Radix Angelicae

			Sinensis
广木香	Guang Mu Xiang	Saussurea root	Radix Saussureae
沉香	Chen Xiang	Aquilaria wood	Lignum Aquilariae Resinatum
茯苓	Fu Ling	Poria	Poria
薏苡仁	Yi Yi Ren	Coix seed	Semen Coicis

·济生肾气丸 Ji-Sheng-Shen-Qi-Wan

Life Preserving Pills for Replenishing Kidney Qi

地黄	Di Huang	Rehmannia root	Radix Rehmanniae
山药	Shan Yao	Chinese yam	Rhizoma Dioscoreae
山茱萸	Shan Zhu Yu	Cornus fruit	Fructus Corni
丹皮	Dan Pi	Mutan bark	Cortex Moutan Radicis
茯苓	Fu Ling	Poria	Poria
泽泻	Ze Xie	Alisma tuber	Rhizoma Alismatis
炮附子	Pao Fu Zi	Prepared aconite root	Radix Aconiti Lateralis Preparata
桂枝	Gui Zhi	Cinnamon twig	Ramulus Cinnamomi
牛膝	Niu Xi	Achryranthes root	Radix Achyranthis Bidentatae
车前子	Che Qian Zi	Plantago seed	Semen Plantaginis

·连朴饮 Lian-Po-Yin

Coptis and Magnolia Decotion

黄连	Huang Lian	Coptis root and rhizome	Rhizoma Coptidis
厚朴	Hou Po	Magnolia bark	Cortex Magnoliae Officinalis
栀子	Zhi Zi	Gardenia fruit	Fructus

			Gardeniae
豆豉	Dou Chi	Prepared soybean	Semen Sojae Praepartatum
半夏	Ban Xia	Pinellia	Rhizoma Pinelliae
芦根	Lu Gen	Phragmites rhizome	Rhizoma Phragmitis
石菖蒲	Shi Chang Pu	Acorus rhizome	Rhizoma Acori Graminei

·六和汤 Liu-He-Tang

Six Harmony Decotion

砂仁	Sha Ren	Cardamon	Fructus Amomi
半夏	Ban Xia	Pinellia	Rhizoma Pinelliae
杏仁	Xing Ren	Apricot seed	Semen Armeniacea Amarum
人参	Ren Shen	Ginseng	Radix Ginseng
白术	Bai Zhu	White atractylodes	Rhizoma Atractylodis Macrocephalae
甘草	Gan Cao	Licorice root	Radix Glycyrrhizae
藿香	Huo Xiang	Agastache	Herba Agastachis
木瓜	Mu Gua	Chaenomeles fruit	Fructus Chaenomelis
厚朴	Hou Po	Magnolia bark	Cortex Magnoliae Officinalis
扁豆	Bian Dou	Dolichos seed	Semen Dolichi
赤茯苓	Chi Fu Ling	Poria	Poria

·六君子汤 Liu-Jun-Zi-Tang

Six Gentlemen Decotion

人参	Ren Shen	Ginseng	Radix Ginseng
茯苓	Fu Ling	Poria	Poria
白术	Bai Zhu	White atractylodes	Rhizoma Atractylodis Macrocephalae
炙甘草	Zhi Gan Cao	Prepared licorice root	Radix Glycyrrhizae Preparata
陈皮	Chen Pi	Tangerine peel	Pericarpium Citri Reticulatae

半夏	Ban Xia	Pinellia	Rhizoma Pinelliae

·苓桂甘汤 Ling-Gui-Zhu-Gan-Tang

Decoction of Poria, Bighead Atractylodes, Cinnamom and Licorice

茯苓	Fu Ling	Poria	Poria
桂枝	Gui Zhi	Cinnamon twig	Ramulus Cinnamomi
白术	Bai Zhu	White atractylodes	Rhizoma Atractylodis Macrocephalae
甘草	Gan Cao	Licorice root	Radix Glycyrrhizae

·龙胆泻肝汤 Long-Dan-Xie-Gan-Tang

Decotion of Gentiana for Purging the Liver Fire

龙胆草	Long Dan Cao	Gentian	Radix Gentianae
柴胡	Chai Hu	Bupleurum root	Radix Bupleuri
黄芩	Huang Qin	Scutellaria root	Radix Scutellariae
栀子	Zhi Zi	Gardenia fruit	Fructus Gardeniae
当归	Dang Gui	Chinese angelica root	Radix Angelicae Sinensis
生地	Sheng Di	Rehmannia root	Radix Rehmanniae
泽泻	Ze Xie	Alisma tuber	Rhizoma Alismatis
木通	Mu Tong	Akebia stem	Caulis Akebiae
车前子	Che Qian Zi	Plantago seed	Semen Plantaginis

·牵正散 Qian-Zheng-San

Powder for Wry Face

白附子	Bai Fu Zi	Typhonium tuber	Rhizoma Typhonii
僵蚕	Jiang Can	Batryticated silkworm	Bombyx Batryticatus
全蝎	Quan Xie	Scorpion	Scorpio

·清胃散 Qing-Wei-San

Powder for Clearing the Stomach Heat

当归	Dang Gui	Chinese angelica root	Radix Angelicae Sinensis
生地	Sheng Di	Rehmannia root	Radix Rehmanniae
丹皮	Dan Pi	Mutan bark	Cortex Moutan Radicis
升麻	Sheng Ma	Cimicifuga rhizome	Rhizoma

			Cimicifugae
黄连	Huang Lian	Coptis root and rhizome	Rhizoma Coptidis

·清营汤 Qing-Ying-Tang

Decotion for clearing Heat in the Nutrient Phase

犀角	Xi Jiao	Rhinoceros horn	Corn Rhinoceri
生地	Sheng Di	Rehmannia root	Radix Rehmanniae
玄参	Xuan Shen	Scrophularia root	Radix Scrophulariae
竹叶心	Zhu Ye Xin	Bamboo shavings	Folium Bambusae
麦冬	Mai Dong	Ophiopogon root	Radiax Ophiopogonis
丹参	Dan Shen	Salvia root	Radix Salviae Miltiorrhizae
黄连	Huang Lian	Coptis root and rhizome	Rhizoma Coptidis
金银花	Jin Yin Hua	Honeysuckle stem	Flos Lonicerae
连翘	Lian Qiao	Forsythia fruit	Fructus Forsythiae

·清瘟败毒饮 Qing-Wen-Bai-Du-Yin

Antipyretic and Antitoxic Decotion

生石膏	Sheng Shi Gao	Gypsum	Gypsum Fibrosum
生地	Sheng Di	Rehmannia root	Radix Rehmanniae
犀角	Xi Jiao	Rhinoceros horn	Corn Rhinoceri
黄连	Huang Lian	Coptis root and rhizome	Rhizoma Coptidis
栀子	Zhi Zi	Gardenia fruit	Fructus Gardeniae
桔梗	Jie Geng	Platycodon root	Radix Platycodi
黄芩	Huang Qin	Scutellaria root	Radix Scutellariae
知母	Zhi Mu	Anemarrhena rhizome	Rhizoma Anemarrhenae
赤芍药	Chi Shao Yao	Red peony	Radix Paeoniae Rubra
玄参	Xuan Shen	Scrophularia root	Radix Scrophulariae
连翘	Lian Qiao	Forsythia fruit	Fructus Forsythiae
甘草	Gan Cao	Licorice root	Radix Glycyrrhizae
丹皮	Dan Pi	Mutan bark	Cortex Moutan

			Radicis
鲜竹叶	Xian Zhu Ye	Fresh bamboo shavings	Folium Bambusae

·羌活胜湿汤 Qiang-Huo-Sheng-Shi-Tang

Decotion of Notopterygium for Rheumatism

羌活	Qiang Huo	Notopterygium root	Rhizoma seu Radix Notoptergii
独活	Du Huo	Pubescent angelica root	Radix Angelicae Pubescentis
川芎	Chuan Xiong	Ligusticum rhizome	Rhizoma Chuanxiong
蔓荆子	Man Jing Zi	Vitex fruit	Fructus Viticis
甘草	Gan Cao	Licorice root	Radix Glycyrrhizae
防风	Fang Feng	Ledebouriella root	Radix Ledebouriellae
藁本	Gao Ben	Straw weed	Rhizome et Radix Ligustici

·人参败毒饮 Ren-Shen-Bai-Du-Yin

Ginseng Antiphlogistic Powder

人参	Ren Shen	Ginseng	Radix Ginseng
茯苓	Fu Ling	Poria	Poria
川芎	Chuan Xiong	Ligusticum rhizome	Rhizoma Chuanxiong
羌活	Qiang Huo	Notopterygium root	Rhizoma seu Radix Notoptergii
独活	Du Huo	Pubescent angelica root	Radix Angelicae Pubescentis
柴胡	Chai Hu	Bupleurum root	Radix Bupleuri
前胡	Qian Hu	Peudedanum root	Radix Peucedani
枳壳	Zhi Qiao	Bitter orange	Fructus Aurantii
桔梗	Jie Geng	Platycodon root	Radix Platycodi
甘草	Gan Cao	Licorice root	Radix Glycyrrhizae

·三仁汤 San-Ren-Tang

Three Kinds of Kernels Decotion

杏仁	Xing Ren	Apricot seed	Semen Armeniacea Amarum
白豆蔻	Bai Dou Kou	Cluster	Semen Cardamomi Rotundi
薏苡仁	Yi Yi Ren	Coix seed	Semen Coicis
滑石	Hua Shi	Talc	Talcum
竹叶	Zhu Ye	Bamboo shavings	Folium Bambusae
通草	Tong Cao	Akebia stem	Caulis Akebiae
厚朴	Hou Po	Magnolia bark	Cortex Magnoliae Officinalis
制半夏	Zhi Ban Xia	Pinellia	Rhizoma Pinelliae

·三才汤 San-Cai-Tang

Triple Ingredients Decotion

天冬	Tian Dong	Asparagus root	Radix Asparagi
生地	Sheng Di	Rehmannia root	Radix Rehmanniae
人参	Ren Sheng	Ginseng	Radix Ginseng

·桑菊饮 Sang-Ju-Yin

Decotion of Mulberry Leaf and Chrysanthemum

桑叶	Sang Ye	Mulberry branch	Folium Mori
菊花	Ju Hua	Chrysantheum flower	Flos Chrysanthem
杏仁	Xing Ren	Apricot seed	Semen Armeniacea Amarum
连翘	Lian Qiao	Forsythia fruit	Fructus Forsythiae
薄荷	Bo He	Mentha	Herba Menthae
桔梗	Jie Geng	Platycodon root	Radix Platycodi
甘草	Gan Cao	Licorice root	Radix Glycyrrhizae
芦根	Lu Gen	Phragmites rhizome	Rhizoma Phragmitis

·沙参麦冬汤 Sha-Shen-Mai-Dong-Tong

Decotion of Glehnia and Ophiopogon

沙参	Sha Shen	Glehnia root	Radix Glehniae
麦冬	Mai Dong	Ophiopogon root	Radiax

			Ophiopogonis
玉竹	Yu Zhu	Polygonatum rhizome	Rhizoma Polygonati Odorati
甘草	Gan Cao	Licorice root	Radix Glycyrrhizae
桑叶	Sang Ye	Mulberry branch	Folium Mori
扁豆	Bian Dou	Dolichos seed	Semen Dolichi
花粉	Hua Fen	Trichosanthes root	Radix Trichosanthis

·参苏饮 Shen-Su-Yin

Ginseng and Perilla Drink

人参	Ren Shen	Ginseng	Radix Ginseng
苏叶	Su Ye	Perilla leaf	Folium Perillae
葛根	Ge Gen	Pueraria root	Radix Puerariae
前胡	Qian Hu	Peucedanum root	Radix Peucedani
法半夏	Fa Ban Xia	Pinellia	Rhizoma Pinelliae
茯苓	Fu Ling	Poria	Poria
橘红	Ju Hong	Pilose asiabell root	Radix Angelicae Sinensis
甘草	Gan Cao	Licorice root	Radix Glycyrrhizae
桔梗	Jie Geng	Platycodon root	Radix Platycodi
枳壳	Zhi Qiao	Bitter orange	Fructus Aurantii
木香	Mu Xiang	Saussurea root	Radix Saussureae
陈皮	Chen Pi	Tangerine peel	Pericarpium Citri Reticulatae
生姜	Sheng Jiang	Fresh ginger	Rhizoma Zingiberis Recens
大枣	Da Zao	Jujube	Fructus Ziziphus Jujubae

·参苓白术散 Shen-Ling-Bai-Zhu-San

Powder of Ginseng, Poria and Bighead Atractylodes

人参	Ren Shen	Ginseng	Radix Ginseng
茯苓	Fu Ling	Poria	Poria
白术	Bai Zhu	White atractylodes	Rhizoma Atractylodis Macrocephalae
桔梗	Jie Geng	Platycodon root	Radix Platycodi
山药	Shan Yao	Chinese yam	Rhizoma Dioscoreae
甘草	Gan Cao	Licorice root	Radix Glycyrrhizae
白扁豆	Bai Bian Dou	Dolichos seed	Semen Dolichi
莲子肉	Lian Zi Rou	Lotus seed	Semen Nelumbinis
砂仁	Sha Ren	Cardamon	Fructus Amomi
薏苡仁	Yi Yi Ren	Coix seed	Semen Coicis

·四君子汤　Si-Jun-Zi-Tang

Fore Gentlemen Decotion

人参	Ren Shen	Ginseng	Radix Ginseng
白术	Bai Zhu	White atractylodes	Rhizoma Atractylodis Macrocephalae
茯苓	Fu Ling	Poria	Poria
甘草	Gan Cao	Licorice root	Radix Glycyrrhizae

·胜湿汤　Sheng-Shi-Tang

Decotion for Removing Dampness

苍术	Cang Zhu	Atractylodes rhizome	Rhizoma Atractylodis
厚朴	Hou Po	Magnolia bark	Cortex Magnoliae Officinalis
半夏	Ban Xia	Pinellia	Rhizoma Pinelliae
藿香	Huo Xiang	Agastache	Herba Agastachis
陈皮	Chen Pi	Tangerine peel	Pericarpium Citri Reticulatae
甘草	Gan Cao	Licorice root	Radix Glycyrrhizae

生姜	Sheng Jiang	Fresh ginger	Rhizoma Zingiberis Recens

·生脉饮 Sheng-Mai-Yin
Pulse Activating Decotion

人参	Ren Shen	Ginseng	Radix Ginseng
麦冬	Mai Dong	Ophiopogon root	Radiax Ophiopogonis
五味子	Wu Wei Zi	Schisandra fruit	Fructus Schisandrae

·失笑散 Shi-Xiao-San
Wonderfol Powder for Reliving Blood Stagnation

蒲黄	Pu Huang	Cat-tail pollen	Pollen Typhae
五灵脂	Wu Ling Zhi	Trogopterus dung	Faeces Trogopterorum

·天麻钩藤饮 Tian-Ma-Gou-Teng-Yin
Drink of Gastrodia and Uncaria

天麻	Tian Ma	Gastrodia tuber	Rhizoma Gastrodiae
钩藤	Gou Teng	Uncaria stem with hooks	Ramulus Uncariae cum Uncis
生石决明	Sheng Jue Ming	Sea-ear shell	Concha Haliotidis
川牛膝	Chuan Niu Xi	Cyathula root	Radix Cyathulae
桑寄生	Sang Ji Sheng	Loranthus	Ramulus Loranthi
杜仲	Du Zhong	Eucommia bark	Cortex Eucommiae
栀子	Zhi Zi	Gardenia fruit	Fructus Gardeniae
黄芩	Huang Qin	Scutellaria root	Radix Scutellariae
益母草	Yi Mu Cao	Leonurus herb	Herba Leonuri
朱茯神	Zhu Fu Shen	Poria	Poria
夜交藤	Ye Jiao Teng	Fleeceflower stem	Caulis Polygoni Multiflori

·天王补心丹 Tian-Wang-Bu-Xin-Dan
Heaven King Heart-Nourishing Pillets

人参	Ren Shen	Ginseng	Radix Ginseng
玄参	Xuan Shen	Scrophularia root	Radix

			Scrophulariae
丹参	Dan Shen	Salvia root	Radix Salviae Miltiorrhizae
茯苓	Fu Ling	Poria	Poria
五味子	Wu Wei Zi	Schisandra fruit	Fructus Schisandrae
远志	Yuan Zhi	Polygala root	Radix Polygalae
桔梗	Jie Geng	Platycodon root	Radix Platycodi
当归身	Dang Gui Shen	Chinese angelica root	Radix Angelicae Sinensis
天冬	Tian Dong	Asparagus root	Radix Asparagi
麦冬	Mai Dong	Ophiopogon root	Radiax Ophiopogonis
柏子仁	Bai Zhi Ren	Biota seed	Semen Biotae
酸枣仁	Suan Zao Ren	Wild jujube	Semen Ziziphi Spinosae
生地黄	Sheng Di Huang	Rehmannia root	Radix Rehmanniae
辰砂	Chen Sha	Cinnabar	Cinnabaris

·温脾汤 Wen-Pi-Tang

Decotion for Warming Spleen

附子	Fu Zi	Typhonium tuber	Rhizoma Typhonii
人参	Ren Shen	Ginseng	Radix Ginseng
大黄	Da Huang	Rhubarb	Radix et Rhizoma Rhei
甘草	Gan Cao	Licorice root	Radix Glycyrrhizae
干姜	Gan Jiang	Dry ginger	Rhizoma Zingiberis

·温经汤 Wen-Jing-Tang

Decotion for Warming Meridian

吴茱萸	Wu Zhu Yu	Evodia fruit	Fructus Evodiae
当归	Dang Gui	Chinese angelica root	Radix Angelicae Sinensis
芍药	Shao Yao	White peony root	Radix Paeoniae Alba

川芎	Chuan Xiong	Ligusticum rhizome	Rhizoma Chuanxiong
人参	Ren Shen	Ginseng	Radix Ginseng
桂枝	Gui Zhi	Cinnamon twig	Ramulus Cinnamomi
阿胶	E Jiao	Gelatin	Colla Corii Asini
丹皮	Dan Pi	Mutan bark	Cortex Moutan Radicis
生姜	Sheng Jiang	Fresh ginger	Rhizoma Zingiberis Recens
半夏	Ban Xia	Pinellia	Rhizoma Pinelliae
麦冬	Mai Dong	Ophiopogon root	Radiax Ophiopogonis

·胃苓汤 Wei-Ling-Tang

Stomach Decoction with Poria

猪苓	Zhu Ling	Polyporus	Polyporus Umbellatus
泽泻	Ze Xie	Alisma tuber	Rhizoma Alismatis
白术	Bai Zhu	White atractylodes	Rhizoma Atractylodis Macrocephalae
茯苓	Fu Ling	Poria	Poria
桂枝	Gui Zhi	Cinnamon twig	Ramulus Cinnamomi
厚朴	Hou Po	Magnolia bark	Cortex Magnoliae Officinalis
陈皮	Chen Pi	Tangerine peel	Pericarpium Citri Reticulatae
苍术	Cang Zhu	Atractylodes rhizome	Rhizoma Atractylodis
甘草	Gan Cao	Licorice root	Radix Glycyrrhizae
生姜	Sheng Jiang	Fresh ginger	Rhizoma Zingiberis

			Recens
大枣	Da Zao	Jujube	Fructus Ziziphus Jujubae

·**犀角地黄汤** Xi-Jiao-Di-Huang-Tang

Decotion of Rhinoceros Horn and Rehmannia

犀角	Xi Jiao	Rhinoceros horn	Corn Rhinoceri
生地黄	Sheng Di Huang	Rehmannia root	Radix Rehmanniae
芍药	Shao Yao	White peony root	Radix Paeoniae Alba
牡丹皮	Mu Dan Pi	Mutan bark	Cortex Moutan Radicis

·**小柴胡汤** Xiao-Chai-Hu-Tang

Minor Decotion of Bupleurum

柴胡	Chai Hu	Bupleurum root	Radix Bupleuri
黄芩	Huang Qin	Scutellaria root	Radix Scutellariae
人参	Ren Shen	Ginseng	Radix Ginseng
半夏	Ban Xia	Pinellia	Rhizoma Pinelliae
甘草	Gan Cao	Licorice root	Radix Glycyrrhizae
生姜	Sheng Jiang	Fresh ginger	Rhizoma Zingiberis Recens
大枣	Da Zao	Jujube	Fructus Ziziphus Jujubae

·**逍遥散** Xiao-Yao-San

Merry Life Powder

柴胡	Chai Hu	Bupleurum root	Radix Bupleuri
当归	Dang Gui	Chinese angelica root	Radix Angelicae Sinensis
白芍	Bai Shao	White peony root	Radix Paeoniae Alba
白术	Bai Zhu	White atractylodes	Rhizoma Atractylodis Macrocephalae
茯苓	Fu Ling	Poria	Poria

甘草	Gan Cao	Licorice root	Radix Glycyrrhizae
薄荷	Bo He	Mentha	Herba Menthae
生姜	Sheng Jiang	Fresh ginger	Rhizoma Zingiberis Recens

·新加白虎汤 Xin-Jia-Bai-Hu-Tang

White Tiger Decotion with Supplement]

生石膏	Sheng Shi Gao	Gypsum	Gypsum Fibrosum
知母	Zhi Mu	Anemarrhena rhizome	Rhizoma Anemarrhenae
陈仓米	Chen Cang mi	Rice	Semen Oryzae
薄荷	Bo He	Mentha	Herba Menthae
竹叶	Zhu Ye	Bamboo shavings	Folium Bambusae
桑枝	Sang Zhi	Mulberry branch	Ramulus Mori
荷叶	He Ye	Leaf of nelumbo nucifera	Folium Nelumbinis
灯心草	Deng Xin Cao	Rush pith	Medulla Junci

·香砂六君子汤 Xiang-Sha-Liu-Jun-Zi-Tang

Six Gentlemen Decotion with Cyperus and Amomum

人参	Ren Shen	Ginseng	Radix Ginseng
白术	Bai Zhu	White atractylodes	Rhizoma Atractylodis Macrocephalae
茯苓	Fu Ling	Poria	Poria
炙甘草	Zhi Gan Cao	Prepared licorice root	Radix Glycyrrhizae Preparata
陈皮	Chen Pi	Tangerine peel	Pericarpium Citri Reticulatae
半夏	Ban Xia	Pinellia	Rhizoma Pinelliae
香附	Xiang Fu	Cyperus tuber	Rhizoma Cyperi
砂仁	Sha Ren	Cardamon	Fructus Amomi

·泻心汤 Xie-Xin-Tang

Decotion for Dispersing the Heart Fire

黄连	Huang Lian	Coptis root and rhizome	Rhizoma Coptidis
黄芩	Huang Qin	Scutellaria root	Radix Scutellariae

大黄	Da Huang	Rhubarb	Radix et Rhizoma Rhei

·益胃汤 Yi-Wei-Tang

Stomach-Nourishing Decotion

沙参	Sha Shen	Glehnia root	Radix Glehniae
麦冬	Mai Dong	Ophiopogon root	Radiax Ophiopogonis
生地黄	Sheng Di Huang	Rehmannia root	Radix Rehmanniae
玉竹	Yu Zhu	Polygonatum rhizome	Rhizoma Polygonati Odorati
冰糖	Bing Tang	rock	Sugar

·一贯煎 Yi-Guan-Jian

An Ever Effective Decotion

北沙参	Bei Sha Shen	Glehnia root	Radix Glehniae
麦冬	Mai Dong	Ophiopogon root	Radiax Ophiopogonis
当归	Dang Gui	Chinese angelica root	Radix Angelicae Sinensis
生地黄	Sheng Di Huang	Rehmannia root	Radix Rehmanniae
枸杞子	Gou Qi Zi	Wolfberry fruit	Fructus Lycii
川楝子	Chuan Lian Zi	Sichuan chinaberry	Fructus Meliae Toosendan

·异功散 Yi-Gong-San

Marvelous Powder

人参	Ren Shen	Ginseng	Radix Ginseng
茯苓	Fu Ling	Poria	Poria
白术	Bai Zhu	White atractylodes	Rhizoma Atractylodis Macrocephalae
甘草	Gan Cao	Licorice root	Radix Glycyrrhizae
陈皮	Chen Pi	Tangerine peel	Pericarpium Citri Reticulatae

·银翘散 Yin-Qiao-San

Powder of Honeysuckle and Forsythia

连翘	Lian Qiao	Forsythia fruit	Fructus Forsythiae
金银花	Jin Yin Hua	Honeysuckle stem	Flos Lonicerae
苦桔梗	Ku Jie Geng	Platycodon root	Radix Platycodi
薄荷	Bo He	Mentha	Herba Menthae
竹叶	Zhu Ye	Bamboo shavings	Folium Bambusae
生甘草	Sheng Gan Cao	Licorice root	Radix Glycyrrhizae
荆芥穗	Jing Jie Sui	Herb of fineleaf schizonepeta	Herba Schizonepetae
淡豆豉	Dan Dou Chi	Prepared soybean	Semen Sojae Praepartatum
牛蒡子	Niu Bang Zi	Arctium fruit	Fructus Arctii
芦根	Lu Gen	Phragmites rhizome	Rhizoma Phragmitis

·真武汤 Zhen-Wu-Tang

Divine Black Bird Decotion

茯苓	Fu Ling	Poria	Poria
芍药	Shao Yao	White peony root	Radix Paeoniae Alba
白术	Bai Zhu	White atractylodes	Rhizoma Atractylodis Macrocephalae
附子	Fu Zi	Typhonium tuber	Rhizoma Typhonii
生姜	Sheng Jiang	Fresh ginger	Rhizoma Zingiberis Recens

·镇肝熄风汤 Zhen-Gan-Xi-Feng-Tang

Decotion for Subduing the Liver to Stop Wind

怀牛膝	Huai Niu Xi	Achryranthes root	Radix Achyranthis Bidentatae
生代赭石	Sheng Dai Zhe Shi	Hematite	Haematitum
生龙骨	Sheng Long Gu	Dragon,s bone	Os Draconis
生牡蛎	Sheng Mu Li	Oyster shell	Concha Ostreae
延胡	Yan Hu	Corydalis tuber	Rhizoma

			Corydalis
天冬	Tian Dong	Asparagus root	Radix Asparagi
川楝子	Chuan Lian Zi	Sichuan chinaberry	Fructus Meliae Toosendan
生麦芽	Sheng Mai Ya	Germinated barley	Fructus Hordei Germinatus
茵陈	Yin Chen	Evergreen artemisia	Herba Artemisiae Capillaris
甘草	Gan Cao	Licorice root	Radix Glycyrrhizae

·栀子柏皮汤 Zhi-Zi-Bai-Pi-Tang
Gardenia and Phellodendron Decotion

栀子	Zhi Zi	Gardenia fruit	Fructus Gardeniae
黄柏	Huang Bai	Phellodendron bark	Cortex Phellodendri
炙甘草	Zhi Gan Can	Prepared licorice root	Radix Glycyrrhizae Preparata

·朱砂安神丸 Zhu-Sha-An-Shen-Wan
Cinnabar Sedative Pills

朱砂	Zhu Sha	Cinnabar	Cinnabaris
黄连	Huang Lian	Coptis root and rhizome	Rhizoma Coptidis
甘草	Gan Cao	Licorice root	Radix Glycyrrhizae
生地	Sheng Di	Rehmannia root	Radix Rehmanniae
当归	Dang Gui	Chinese angelica root	Radix Angelicae Sinensis

舌象图片（The Tongue Picture）

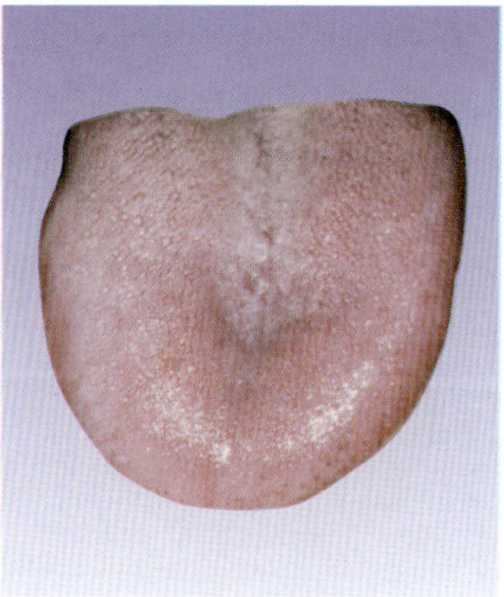

图1.1 有神舌(淡红舌)
Figure 1.1 The Tongue with Spirit (The Light Red Tongue)

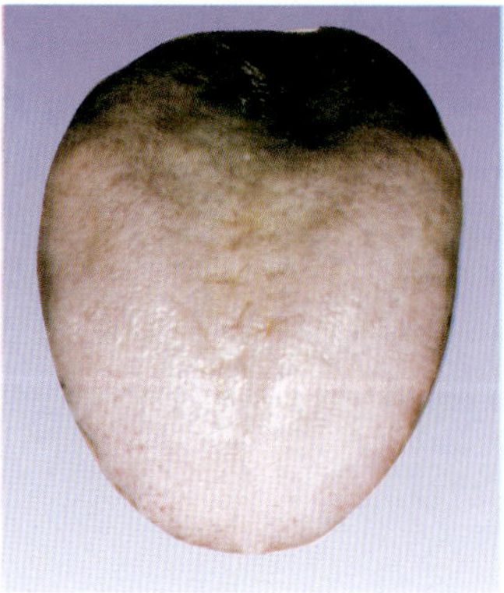

图2.1 淡白舌
Figure 2.1 The Pale Tongue

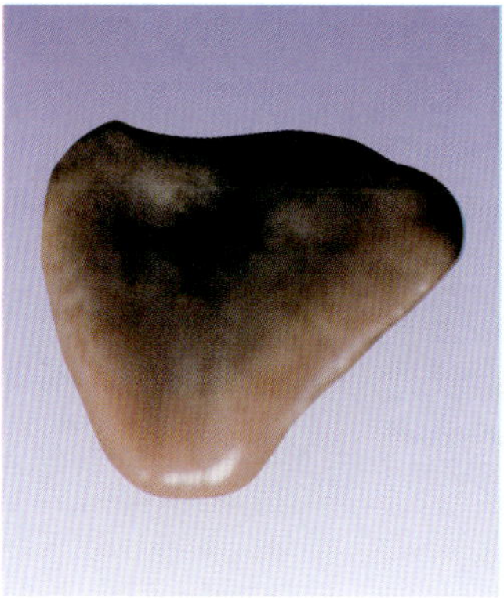

图2.2 淡白瘦薄舌
Figure 2.2 The Thin and Pale Tongue

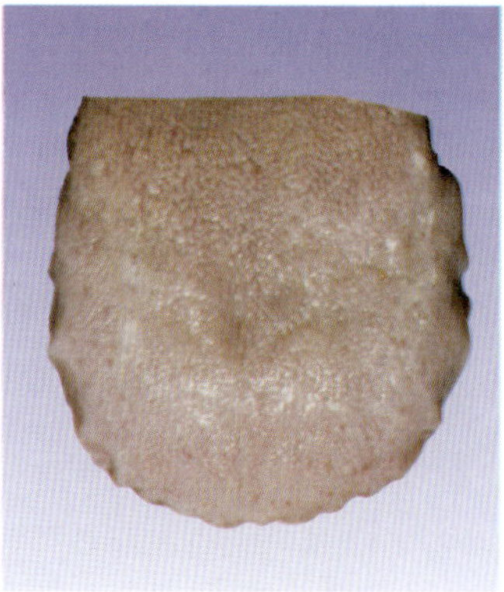

图2.3 淡白胖嫩齿痕舌
Figure 2.3 The Pale, Enlarged and Tender Tongue with Tooth Prints

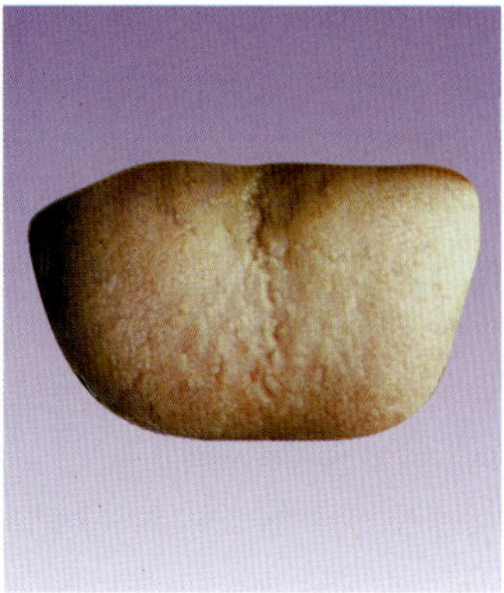

图2.4 淡白舌，白腻干苔
Figure 2.4 The Pale Tongue with Dry, White and Sticky Fur

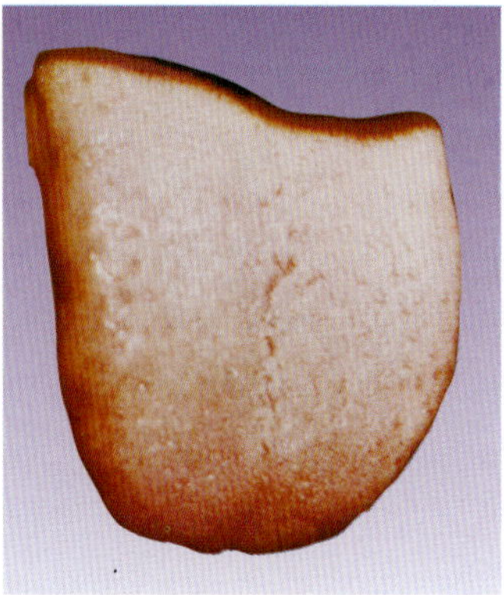

图2.5 淡白夹红舌
Figure 2.5 The Pale Tongue with Red Parts

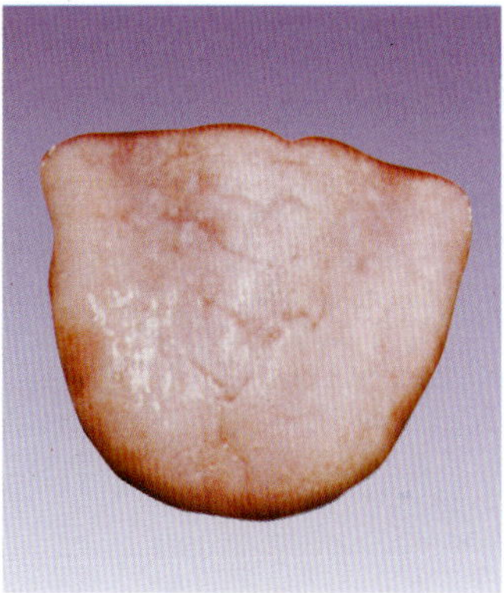

图2.6 淡白光莹舌（枯白舌）
Figure 2.6 The Pale and Glossy Tongue (Withered White Tongue)

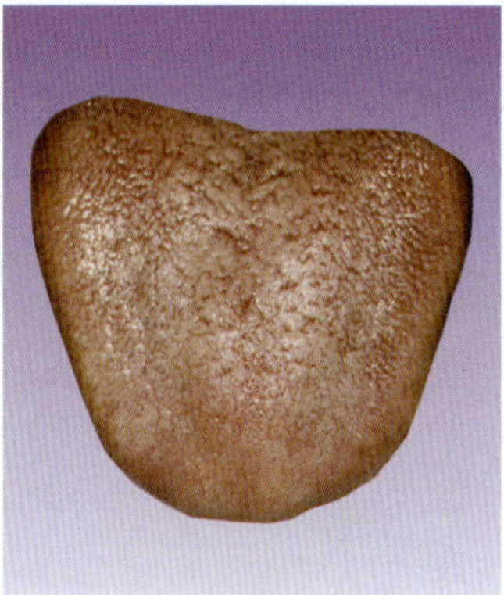

图2.7 淡白偏暗舌
Figure 2.7 The Pale and Dim Tongue

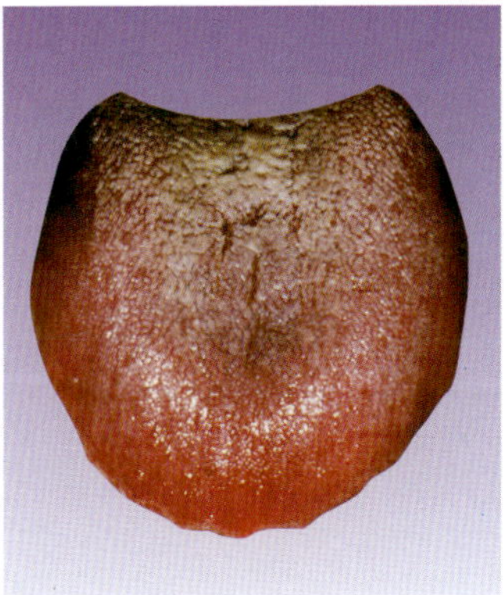

图2.8 红舌
Figure 2.8 The Red Tongue

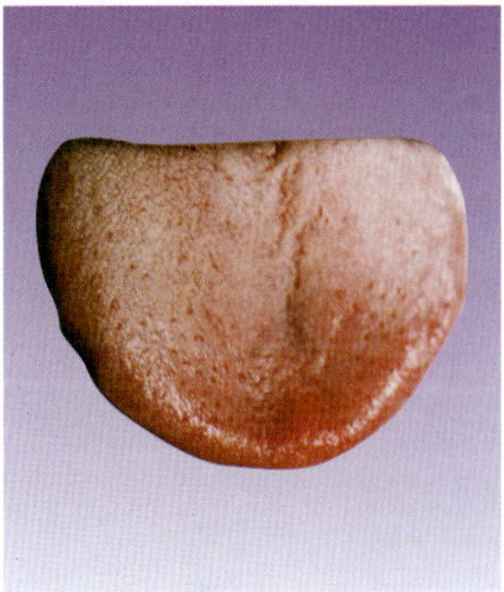

图2.9 舌边尖红（薄白苔）
Figure 2.9 The Tongue With Red Sides and Tip (Thin White Fur)

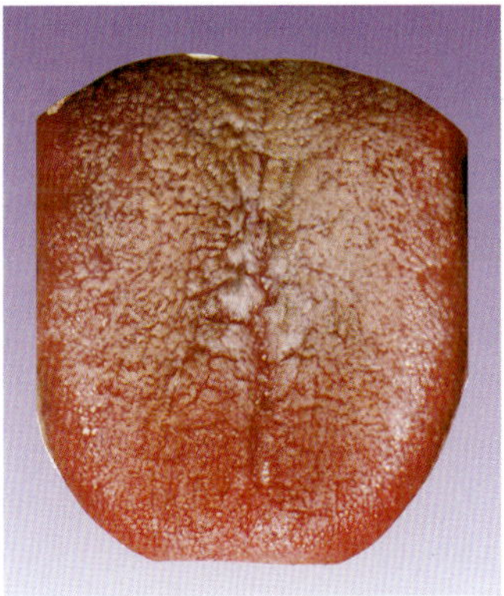

图2.10 舌红（苔黄厚干燥）
Figure 2.10 The Red Tongue (with the Yellow, Thick and Dry Fur)

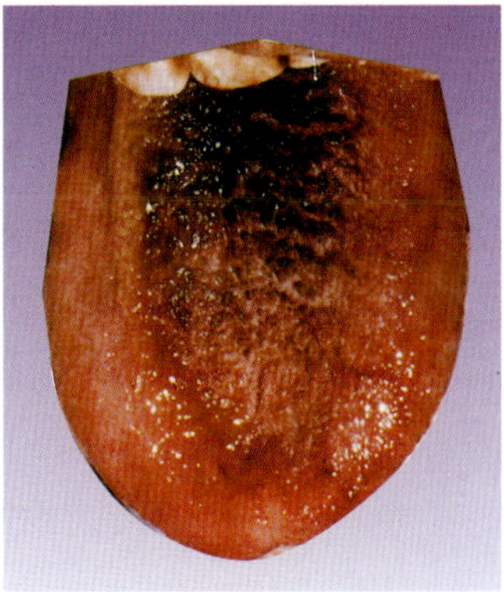

图2.11 舌红偏暗（苔焦黄、灰黑）
Figure 2.11 The Red, Slight Dark Tongue (Covered by Dark Yellow, or Gray Black Fur)

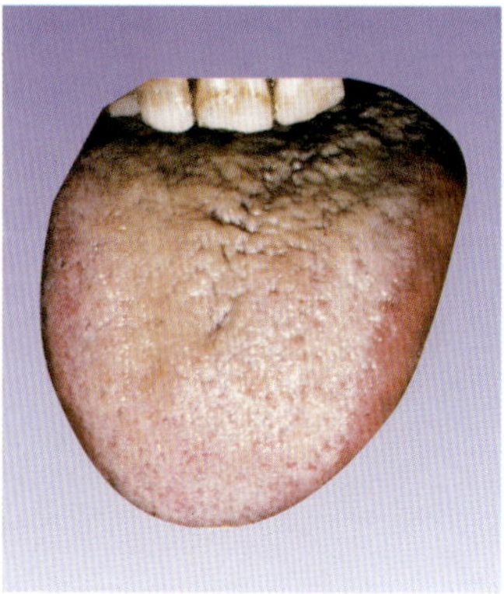

图2.12 舌红（苔黄腻）

Figure 2.12 The Red Tongue (with Yellow and Sticky Fur)

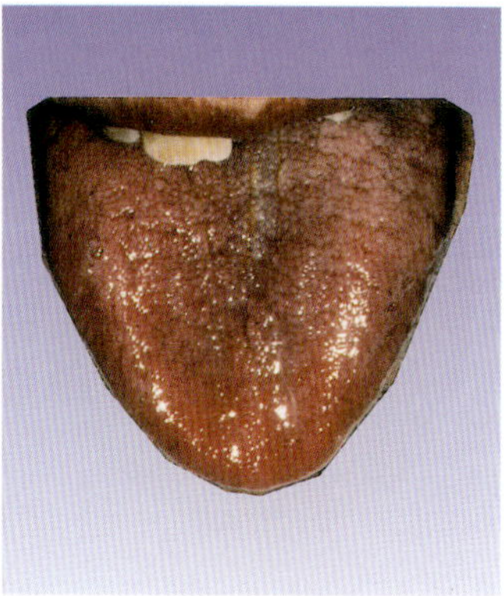

图2.13 舌红（少苔）

Figure 2.13 The Red Tongue (with Less Fur)

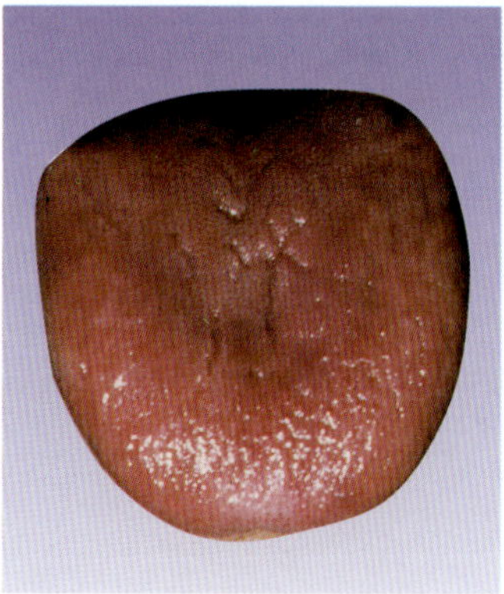

图2.14 绛舌少苔

Figure 2.14 The Crimson Tongue with Less Fur

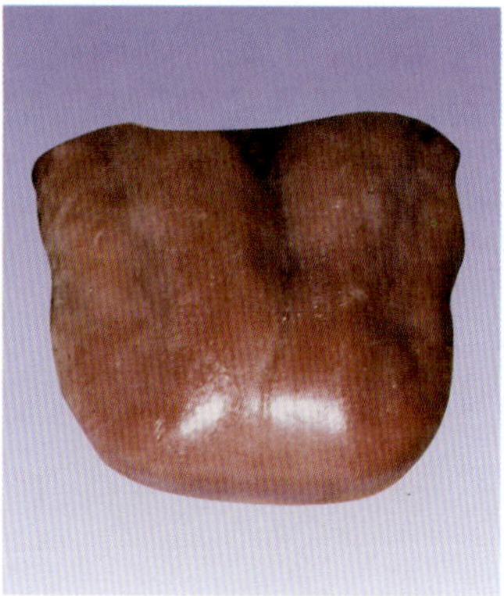

图2.15 红绛光莹舌

Figure 2.15 The Crimson and Golssy Tongue

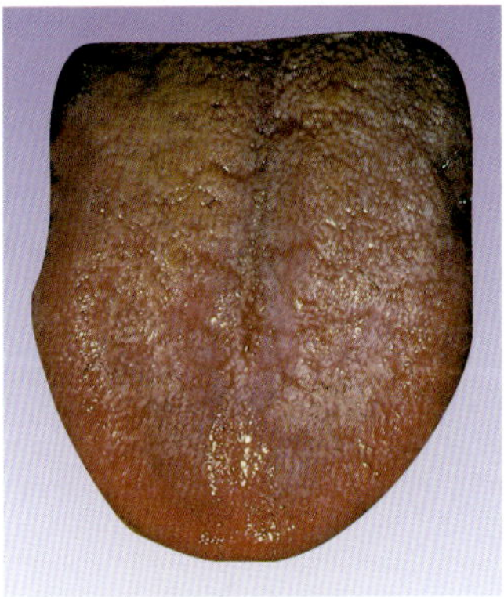

图 2.16 红绛晦暗枯瘦舌

Figure 2.16 The Dark Crimson and Emaciated Tongue

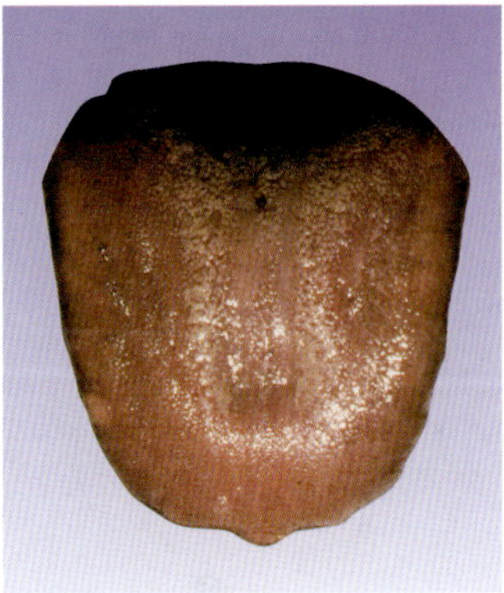

图 2.17 紫绛舌

Figure 2.17 The Purple-Crimson Tongue

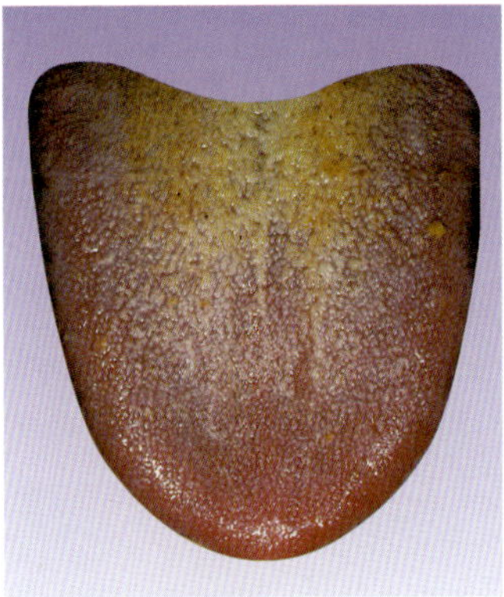

图 2.18 紫晦舌

Figure 2.18 The Crimson and Dim Tongue

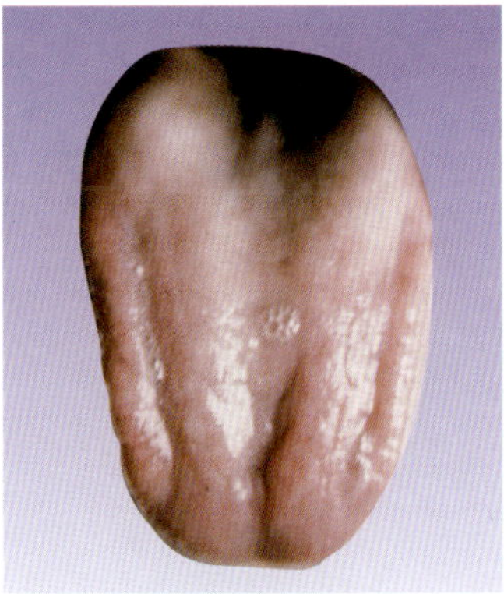

图 2.19 淡白青紫舌

Figure 2.19 The Pale and Bluish Purple Tongue

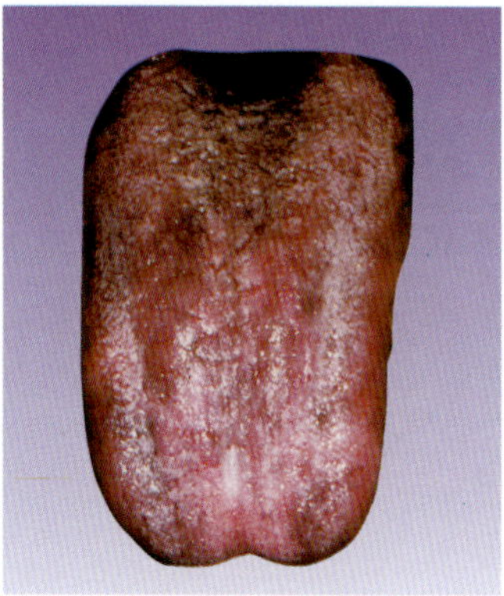

图2.20 紫暗瘀斑瘀点舌
Figure 2.20 The Dark Purple Tongue with Blue Spots

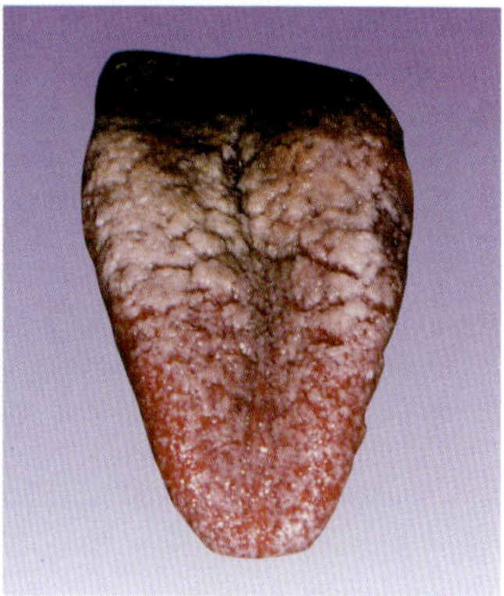

图3.1 苍老舌
Figure 3.1 The Bleak and Dark Tongue

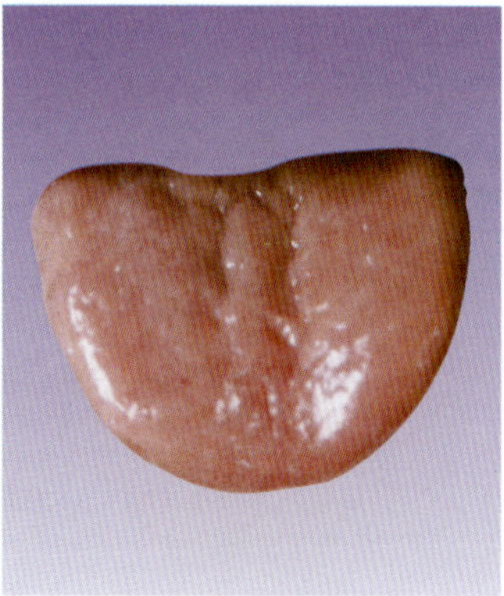

图3.2 娇嫩舌（淡白）
Figure 3.2 The Tender Tongue (Pale)

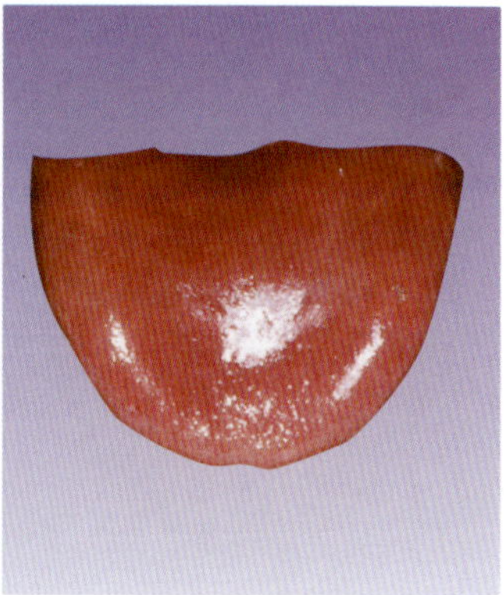

图3.3 娇嫩舌(色红)
Figure 3.3 The Tender Tongue (Fresh Red)

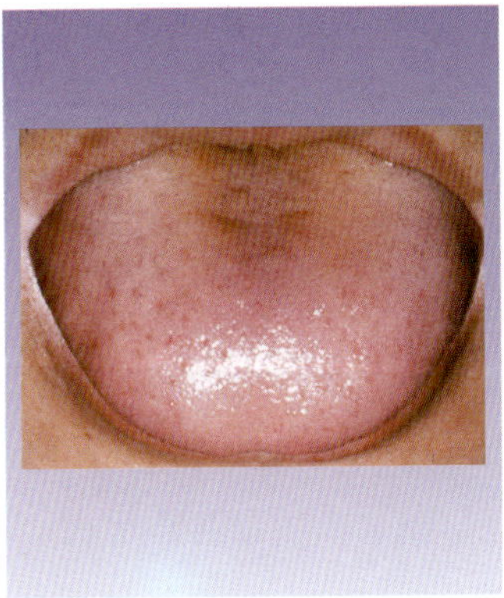

图3.4 胖大舌

Figure 3.4 The Big and Fat Tongue

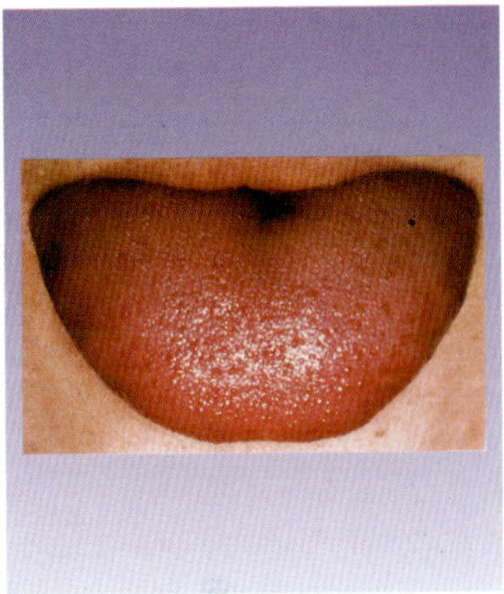

图3.5 鲜红肿胀舌

Figure 3.5 The Fresh Red Swollen Tongue

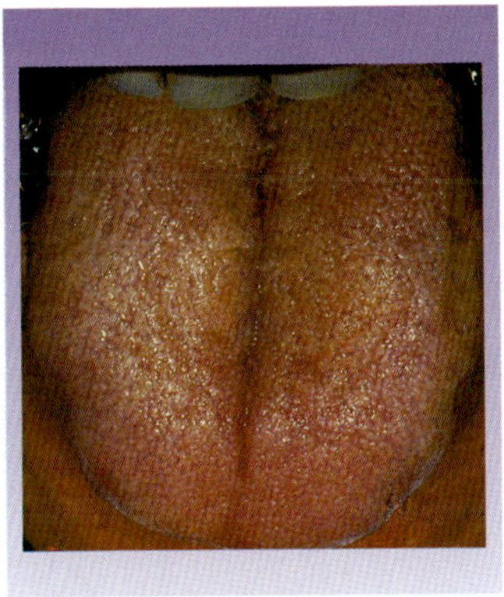

图3.6 青紫肿胀舌

Figure 3.6 The Swollen Tongue in Black Purple Color

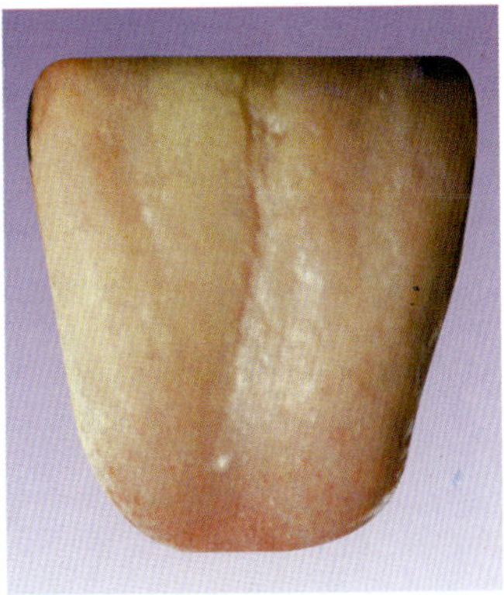

图3.7 淡白瘦薄舌

Figure 3.7 The Thin and Small Tongue in Light White Color

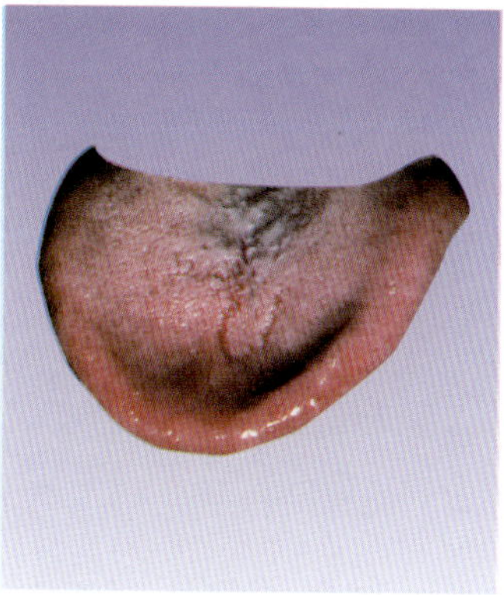

图 3.8 红绛瘦薄舌

Figure 3.8 The Thin and Small Tongue in Red and Dark Purple Color

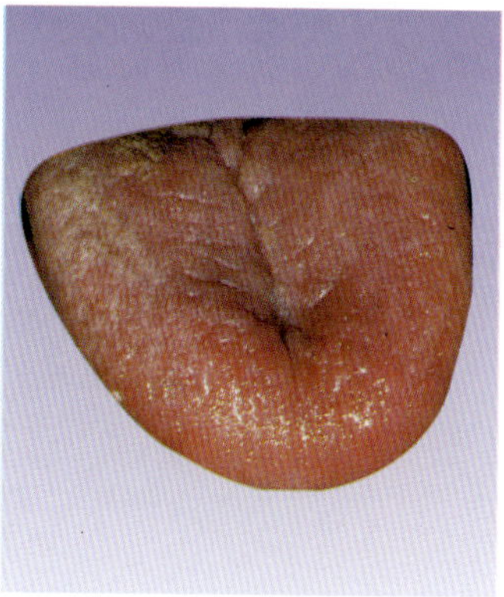

图 3.9 红绛少苔裂纹舌

Figure 3.9 The Fissure Tongue in Red and Crimson Color, with Less Fur

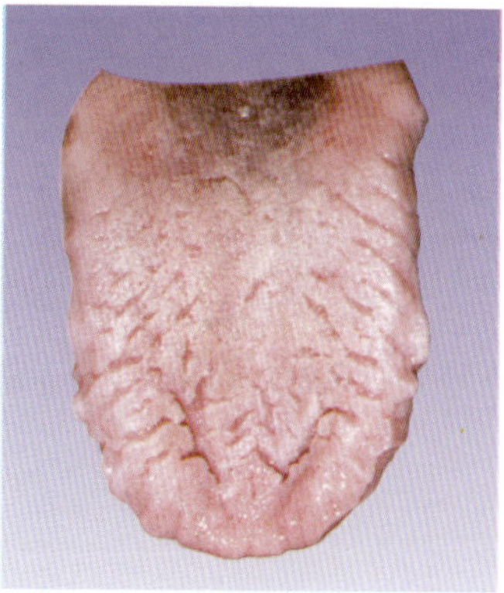

图 3.10 淡白裂纹舌

Figure 3.10 The Fissure Tongue in Pale Color

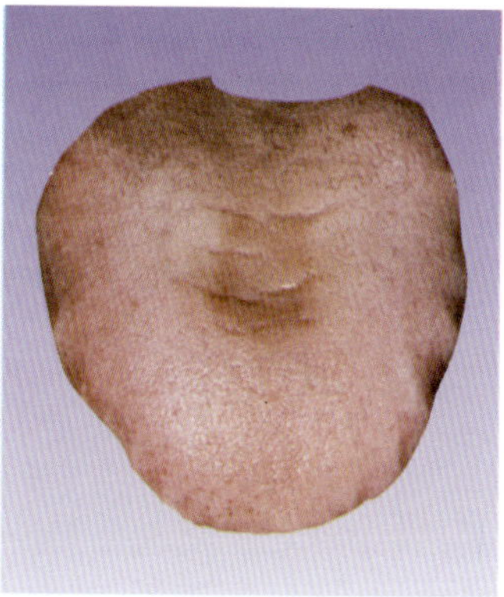

图 3.11 齿痕舌

Figure 3.11 The Tongue with Tooth Prints

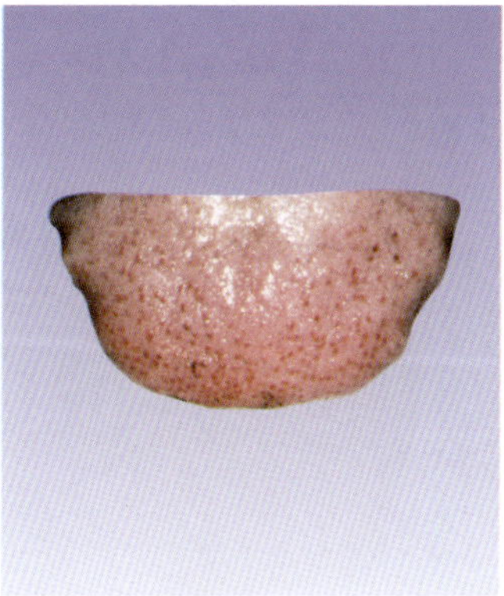

图 3.12 点刺舌
Figure 3.12 The Dot and Thorn Tongue

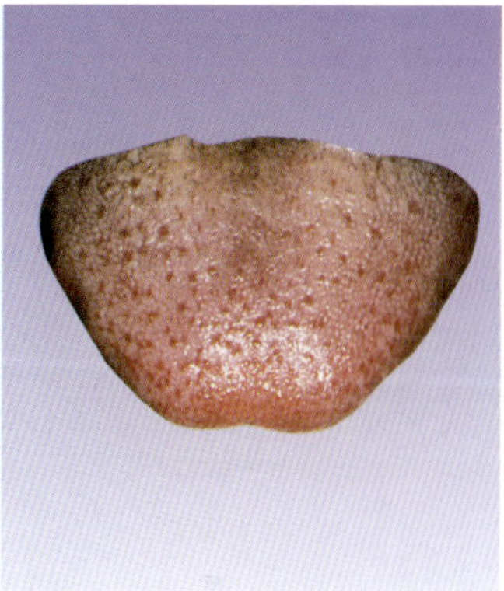

图 3.13 红绛芒刺舌（杨梅舌）
Figure 3.13 The Thorny Tongue in Red and Crimson Color (Bayberry or Strawberry Tongue)

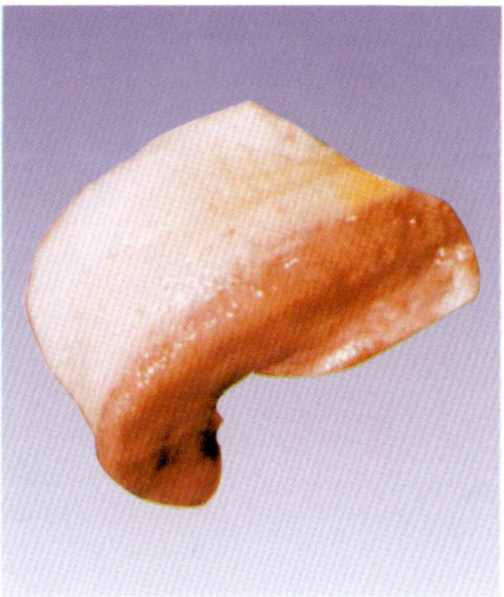

图 3.14 重舌
Figure 3.14 The Double Tongue

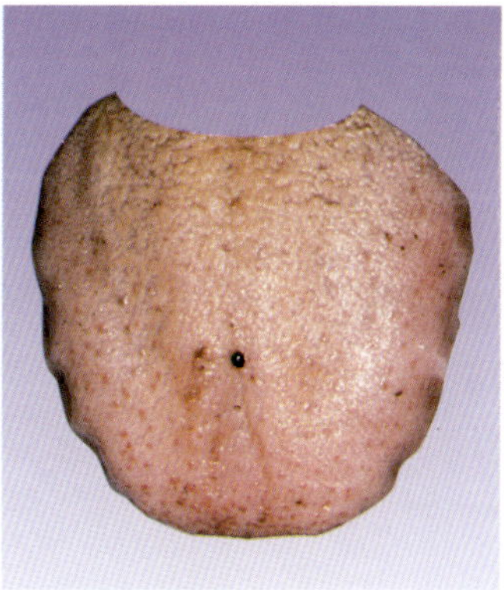

图 3.15 舌衄
Figure 3.15 The Bleeding Tongue

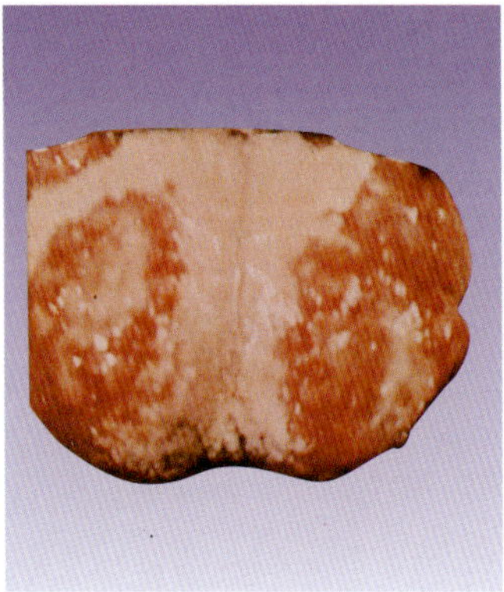

图 3.16 舌痈

Figure 3.16 Abscess of the Tongue

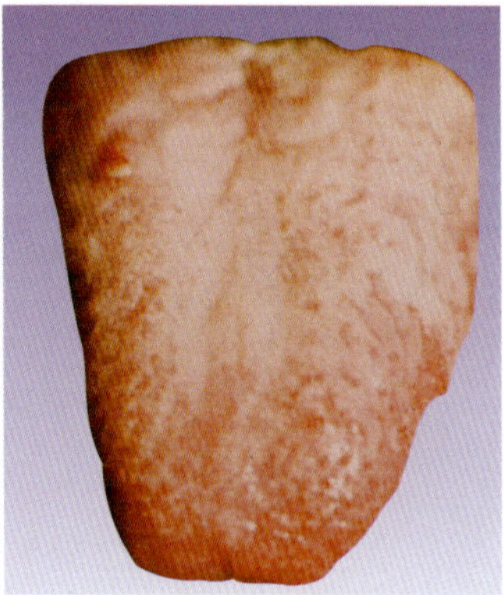

图 3.17 舌疔

Figure 3.17 The Tongue Pustule

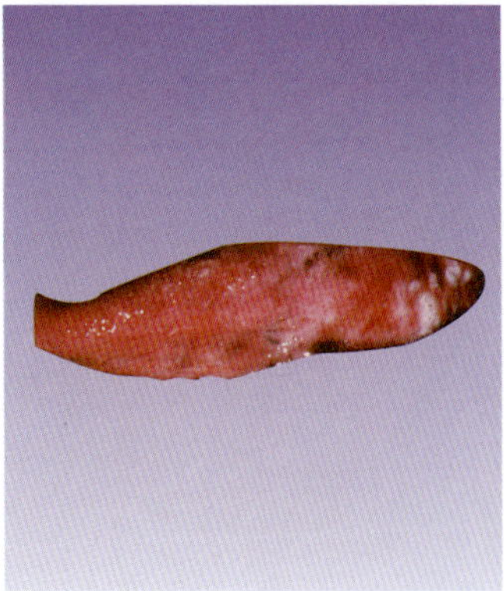

图 3.18 舌疮

Figure 3.18 Boils of Tongue

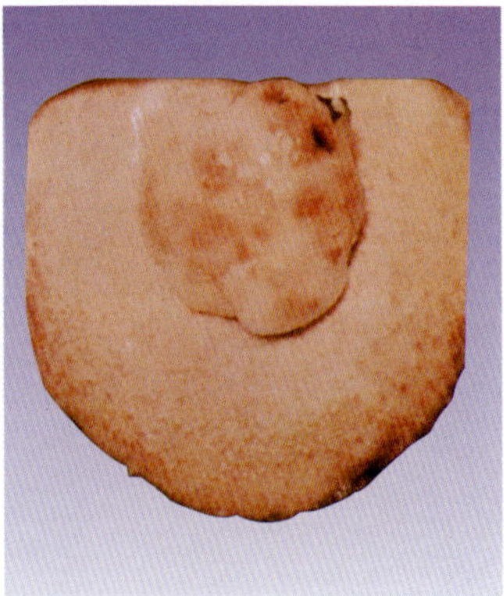

图 3.19 舌菌

Figure 3.19 The Carcinoma of the Tongue

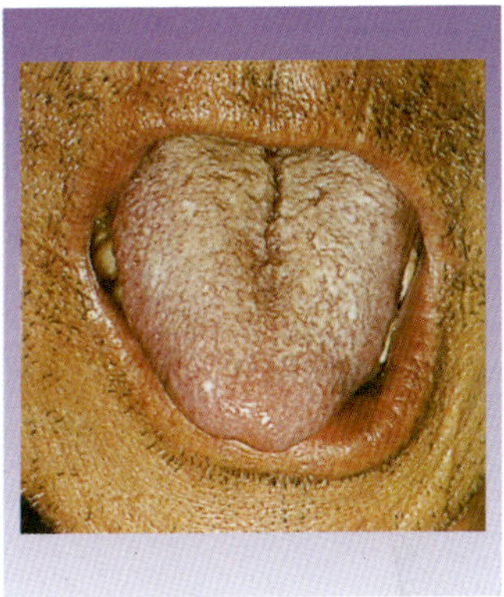

图4.1 强硬舌

Figure 4.1 The Stiff Tongue

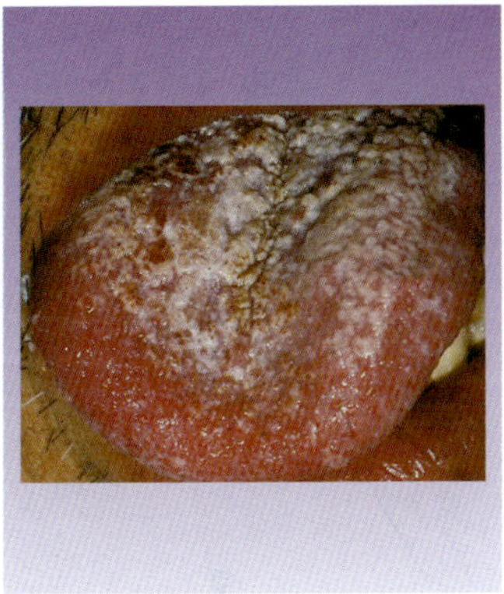

图4.2 歪斜舌

Figure 4.2 The Deviated Tongue

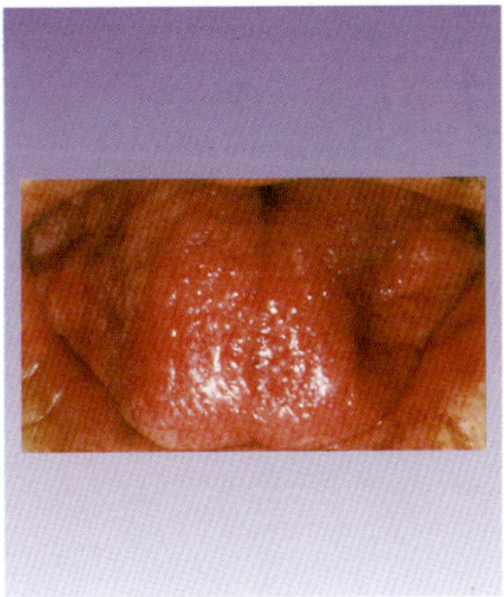

图4.3 短缩舌

Figure 4.3 The Shortened and Retracted Tongue

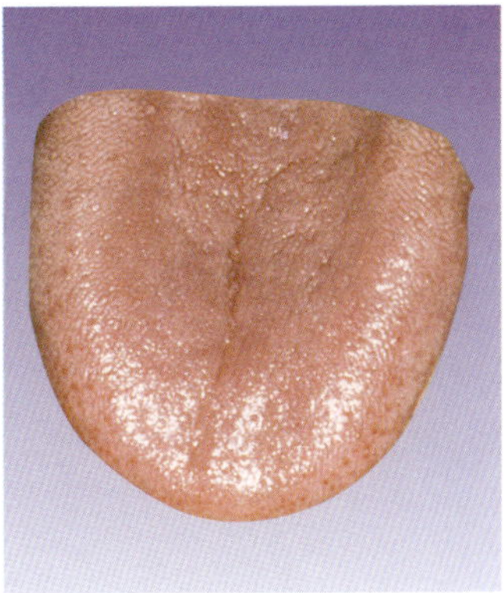

图5.1 薄苔（润苔）

Figure 5.1 Thin Coating (Moist Coating)

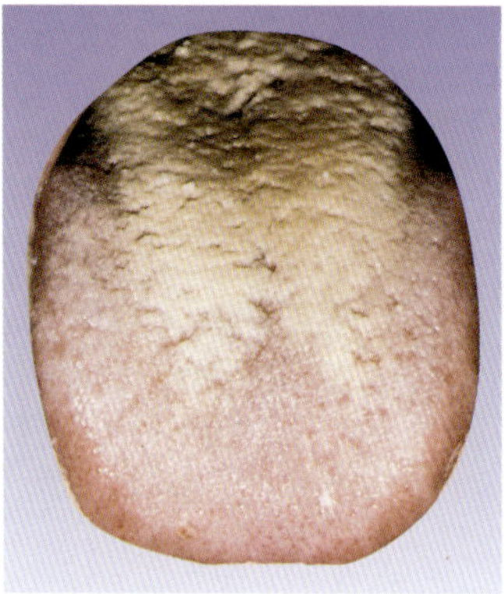

图5.2 厚苔
Figure 5.2 Thick Coating

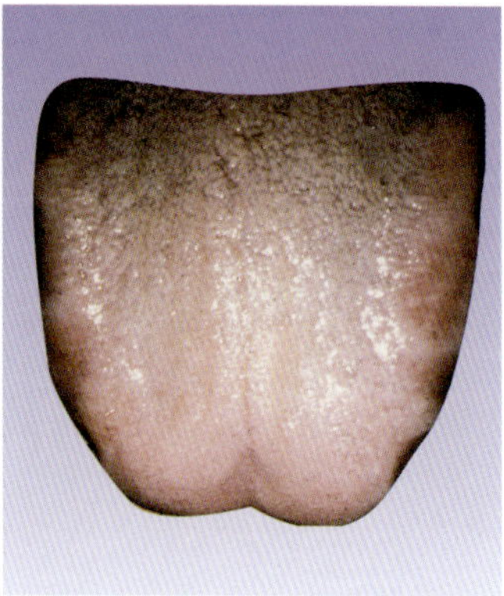

图5.3 滑苔
Figure 5.3 Watery Coating

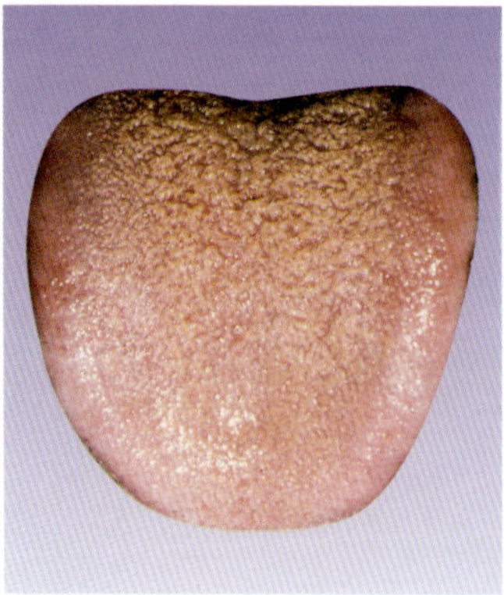

图5.4 糙苔
Figure 5.5 Rough Coating

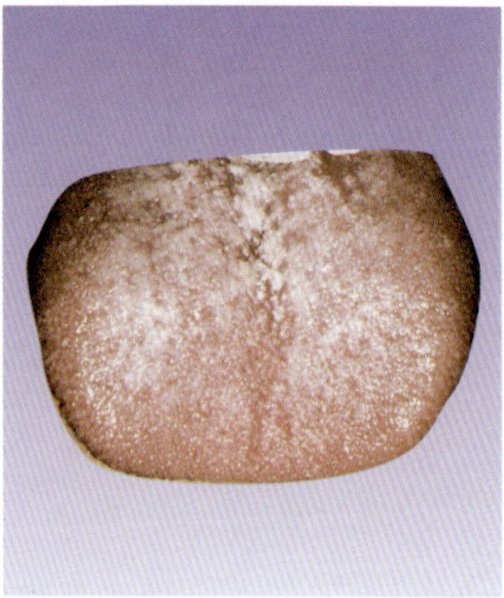

图5.5 腐苔
Figure 5.5 Curdy Coating

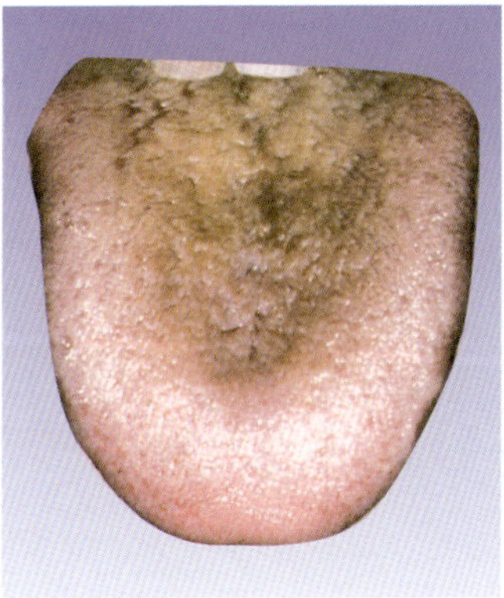

图5.6 腻苔

Figure 5.6 Sticky Coating

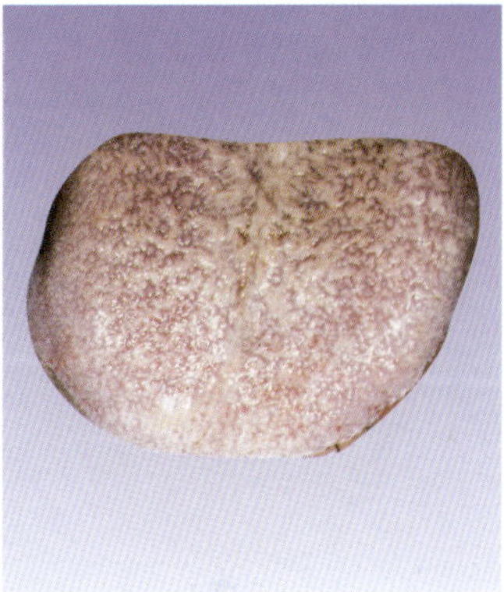

图5.7 全（苔）

Figure 5.7 Full Coating

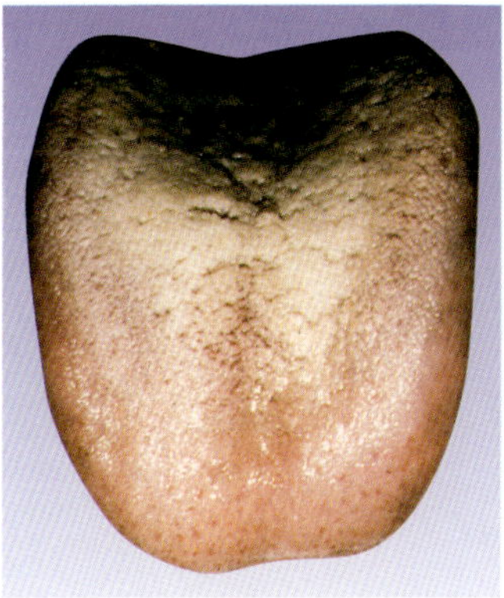

图5.8 偏（苔）

Figure 5.8 Partial Coating

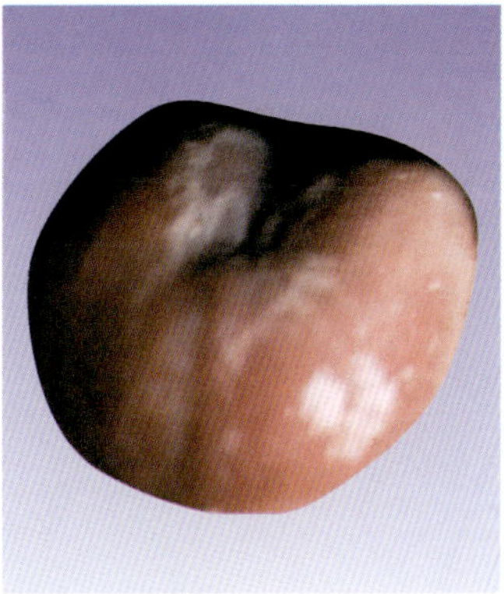

图5.9 花剥苔

Figure 5.9 The Exfoliated Fur

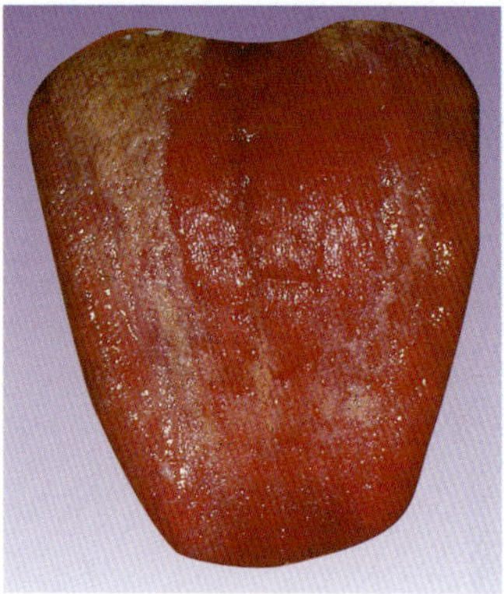

图5.10 地图舌

Figure 5.10 The Map Tongue

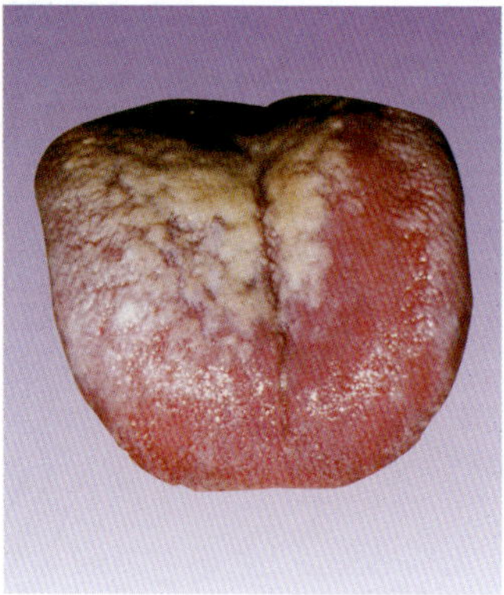

图5.11 类剥苔

Figure 5.11 The Exfoliative kind of Coating

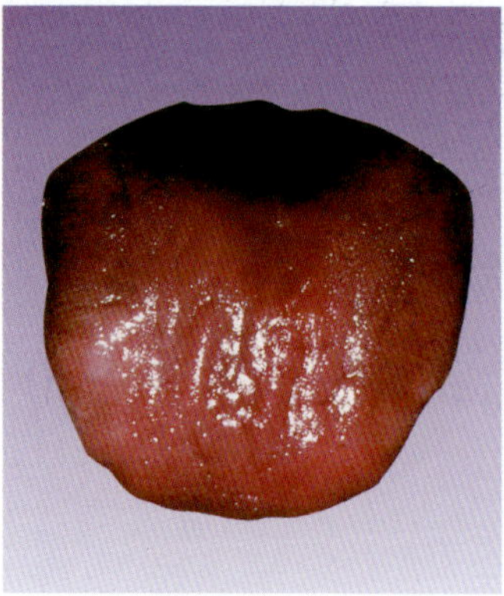

图5.12 镜面舌

Figure 5.12 The Mirror-like Tongue

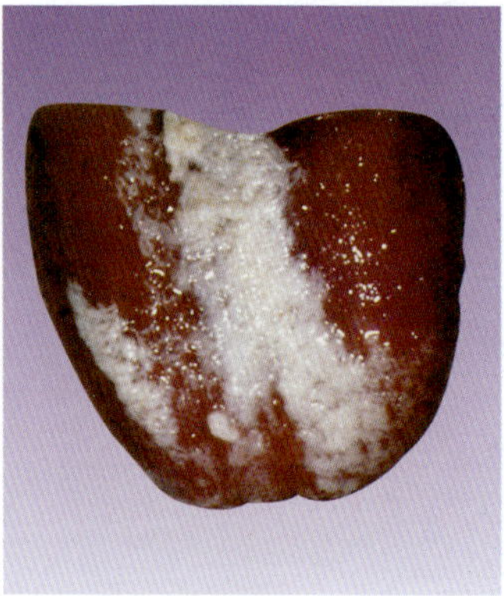

图5.13 无根假苔

Figure 5.13 False Fur without any Root

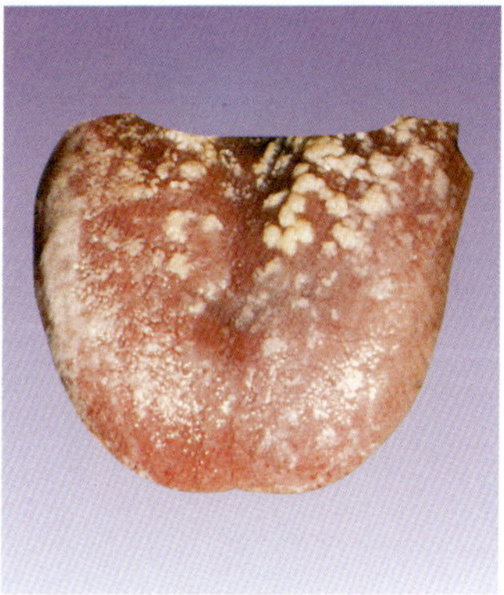

图5.14 无根浮垢苔

Figure 5.14 The Loosely Dirty Fur without any Root

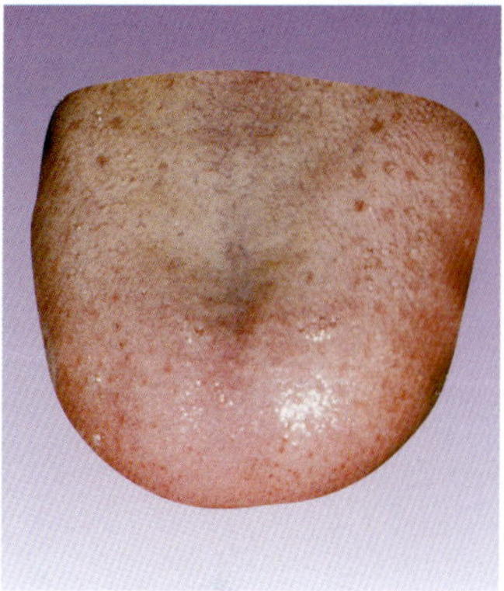

图6.1 薄白苔

Figure 6.1 The Thin and White Coating

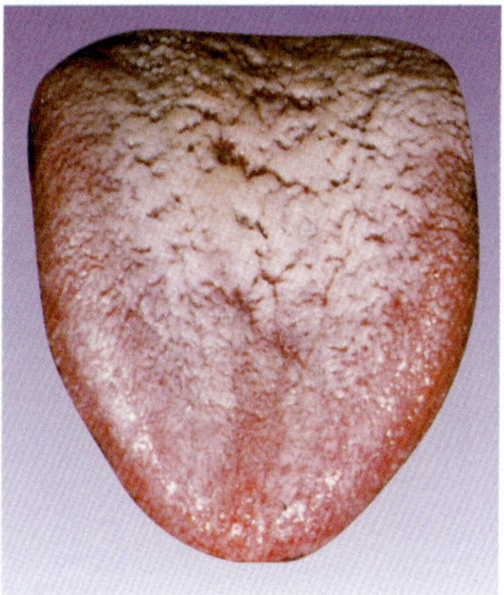

图6.2 白厚苔

Figure 6.2 The Thick and White Coating

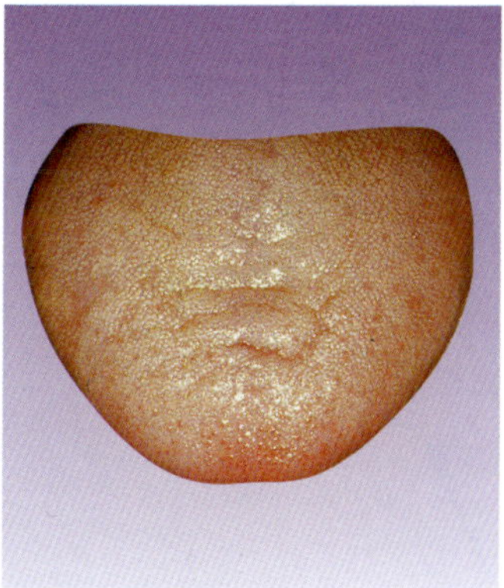

图6.3 白滑苔

Figure 6.3 The Watery and White Coating

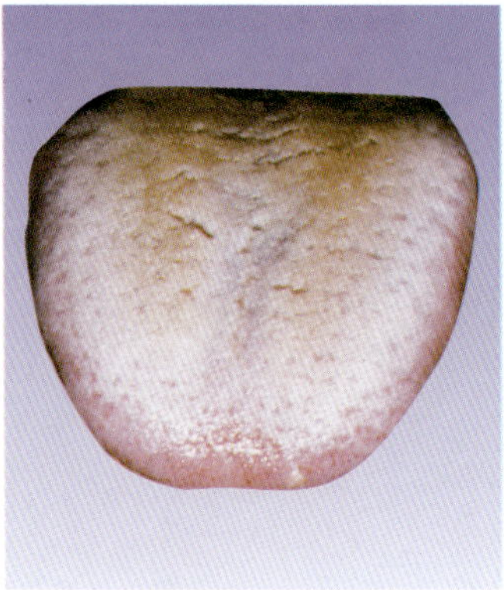

图6.4 白腻苔
Figure 6.4 The White Greasy Coating

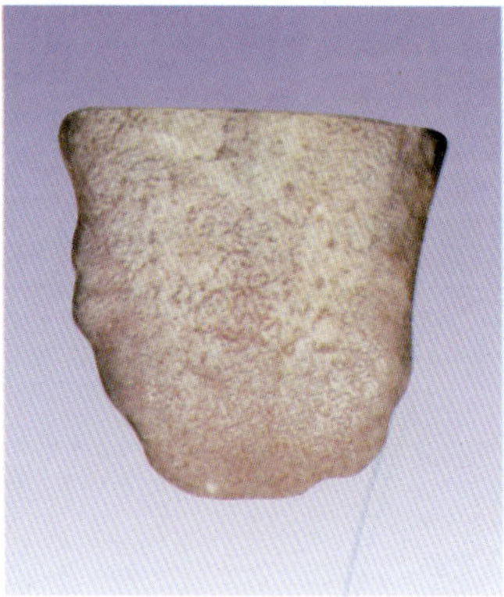

图6.5 白腻干苔
Figure 6.5 The Dry and White Greasy Coating

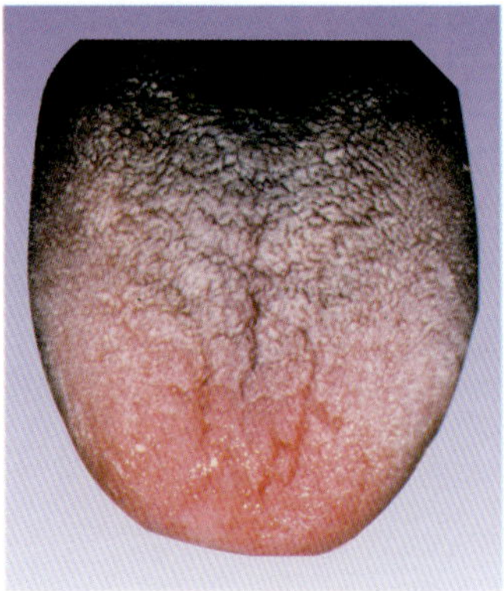

图6.6 白糙、裂苔（白砂苔）
Figure 6.6 The White Tough and Split Coating (white and coating)

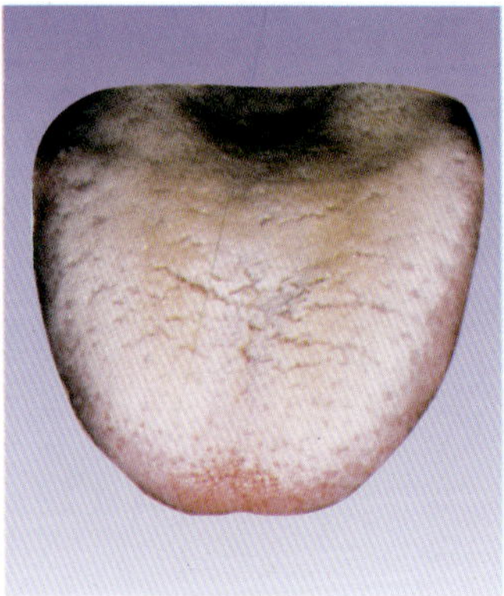

图6.7 白如积粉苔
Figure 6.7 The White Powder Coating

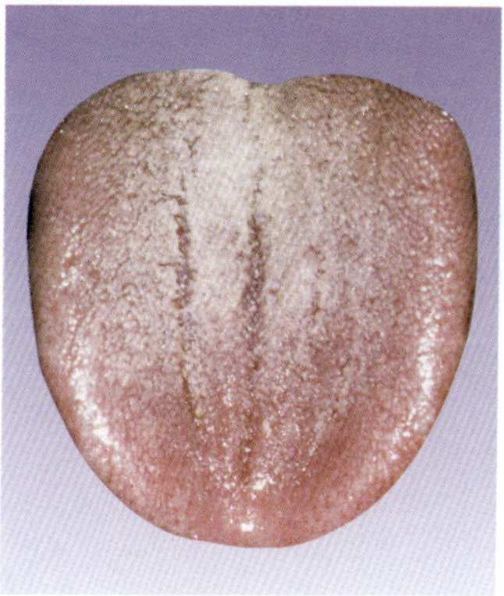

图6.8 薄黄苔

Figure 6.8 The Thin and Yellow Coating

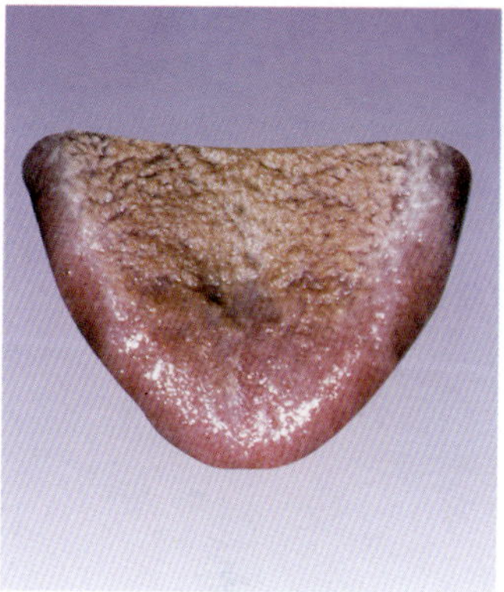

图6.9 黄厚（燥）苔

Figure 6.9 The Thick, Dry and Yellow Coating

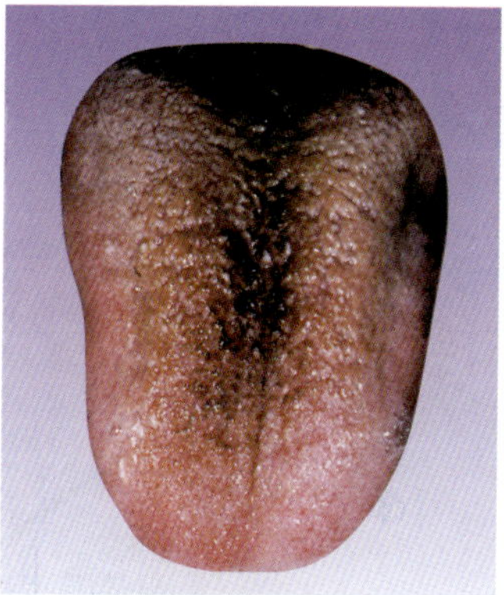

图6.10 焦黄苔

Figure 6.10 The Black Yellow Coating

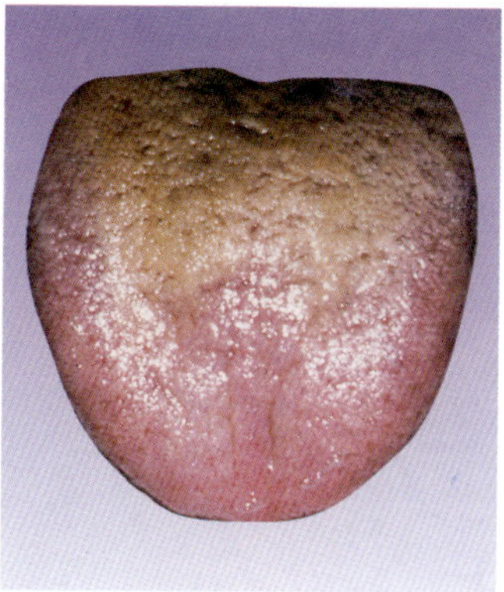

图6.11 黄腻苔

Figure 6.11 The Yellow and Greasy Coating

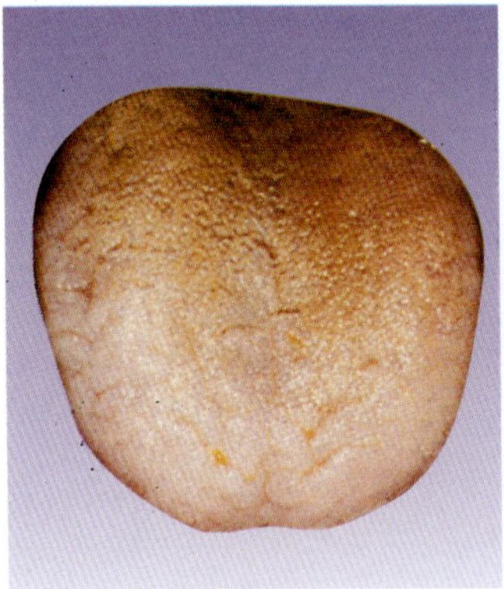

图6.12 淡黄滑苔
Figure 6.12 The Light Yellow and Watery Coating

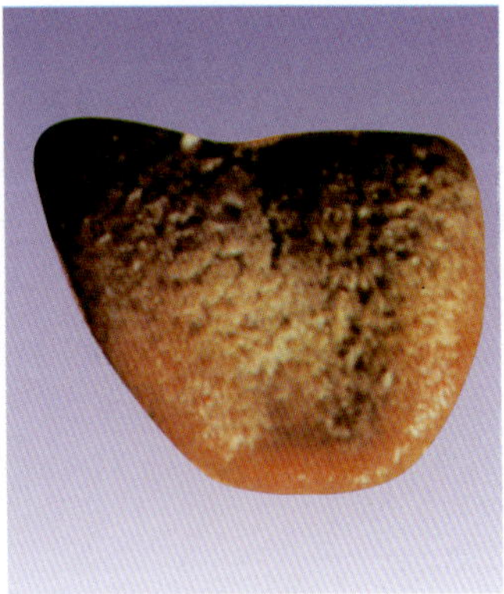

图6.13 焦黑干燥苔
Figure 6.13 Dry and Black Coating

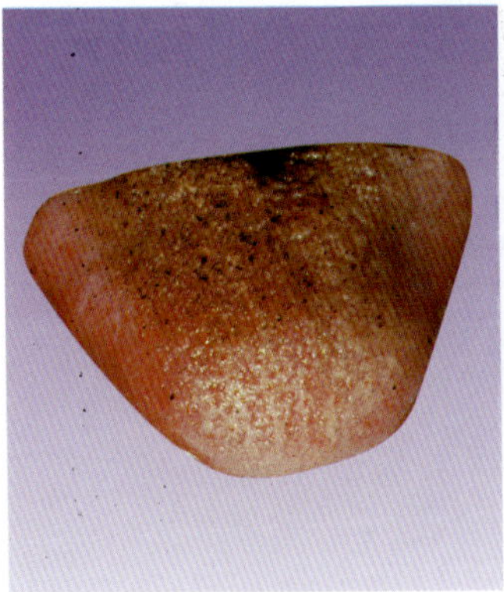

图6.14 白腻灰黑苔
Figure 6.14 The White Greasy and Gray Darkness Coating

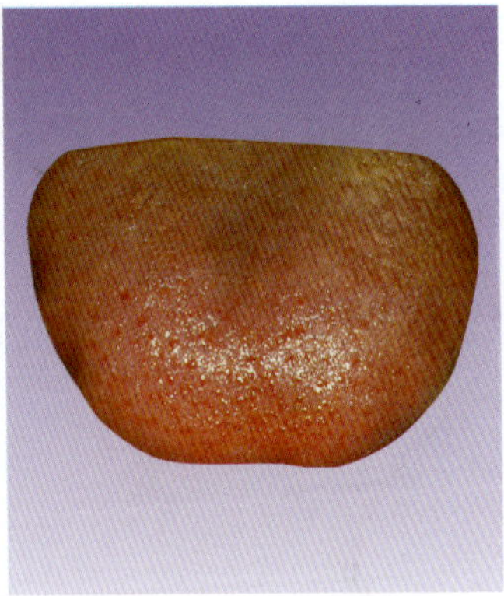

图7.1 淡白红点舌，薄白苔
Figure 7.1 The Pale Tongue with Red Spots, Covered by Thin White Fur

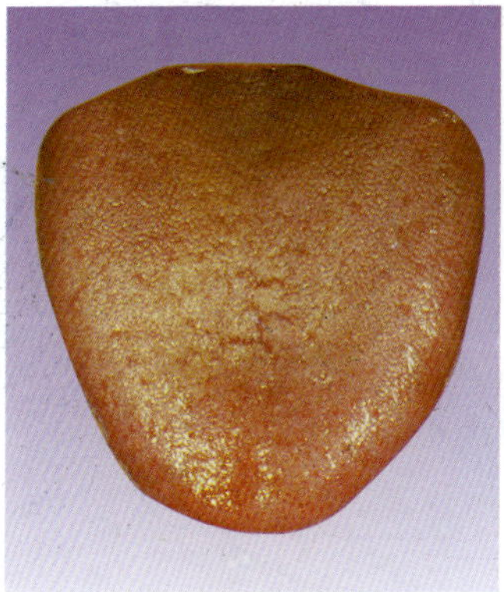

图7.2 淡白舌，薄白腻苔
Figure 7.2 The Pale Tongue Covered with Thin, White and Sticky Fur

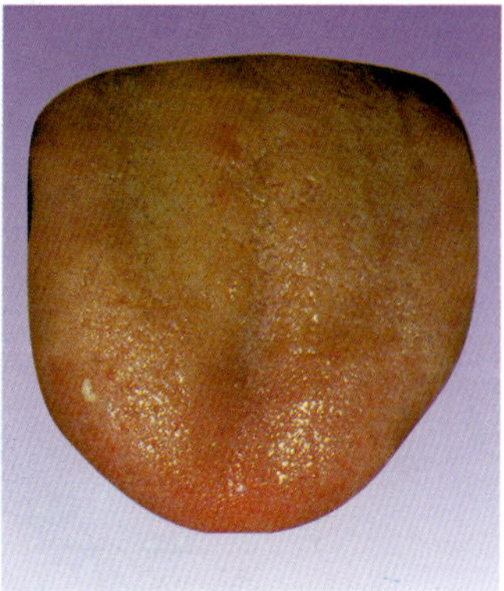

图7.3 淡白舌，白滑苔
Figure 7.3 The Pale Tongue with White and Watery Coating

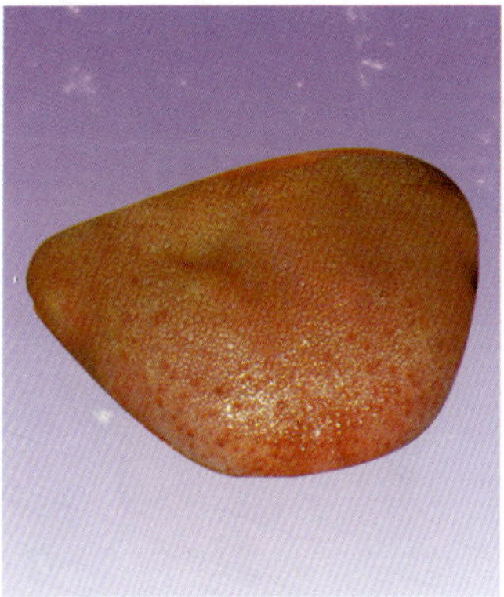

图7.4 淡白黑点舌，薄白根腻苔
Figure 7.4 The Pale Tongue with Black Spots, Covered by Thin White Fur as well as Sticky Fur Seen at the Root

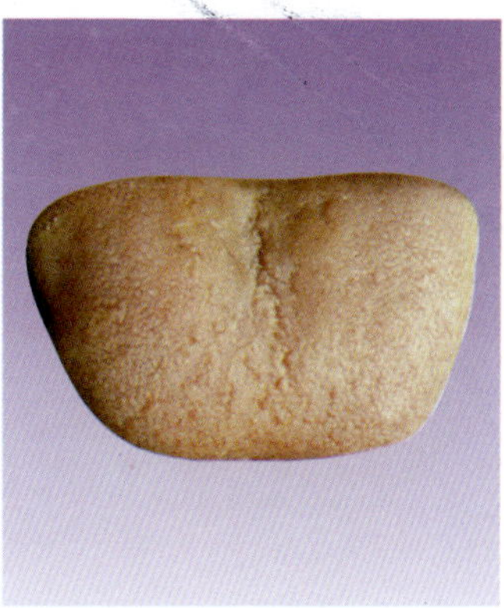

图7.5 淡白舌，白厚苔
Figure 7.5 The Pale Tongue with White and Thick Fur

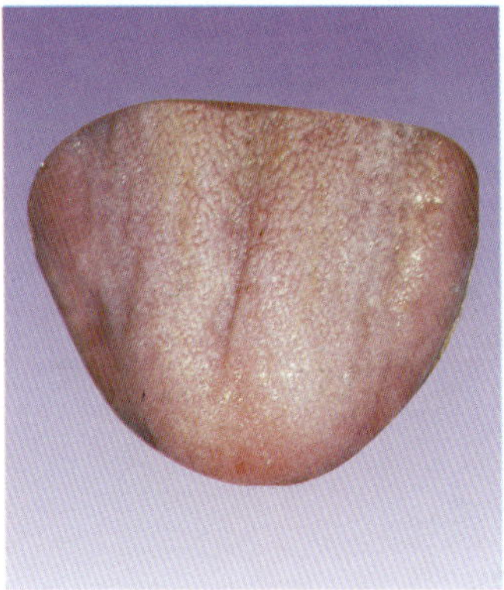

图7.6 淡白略暗舌，薄白淡黄苔

Figure 7.6 The Pale and Dim Tongue Covered by the Thin White and Light Yellow Coating

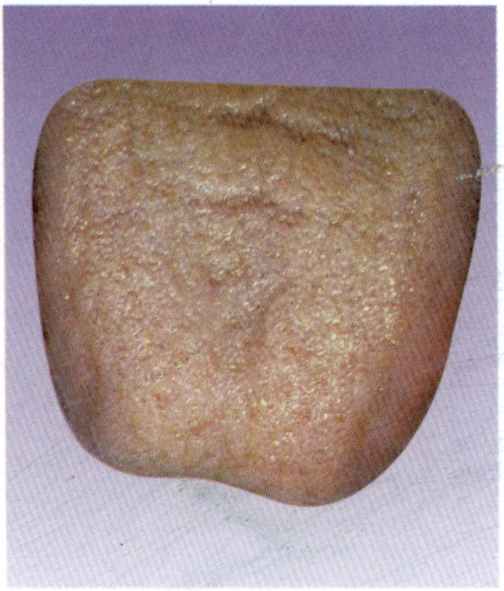

图7.7 淡白偏暗舌，薄白根黄苔

Figure 7.7 The Pale Dark Tongue Covered by Thin White Fur with Yellow Color at the Root

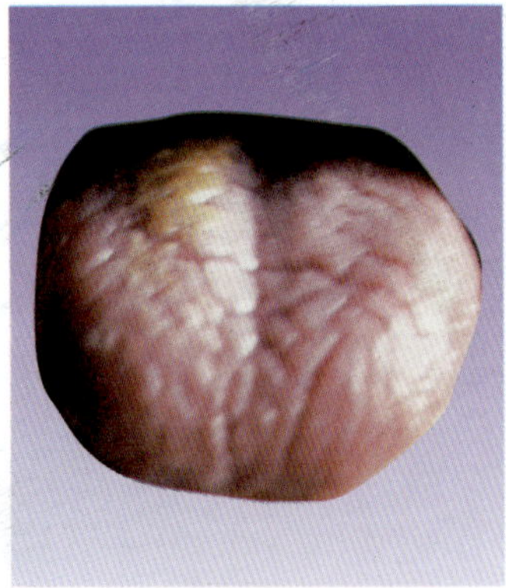

图7.8 淡白裂纹舌，偏黄浮垢苔

Figure 7.8 The Pale and Fissured Tongue with a Layer of Yellow, Floating and Turbid Fur

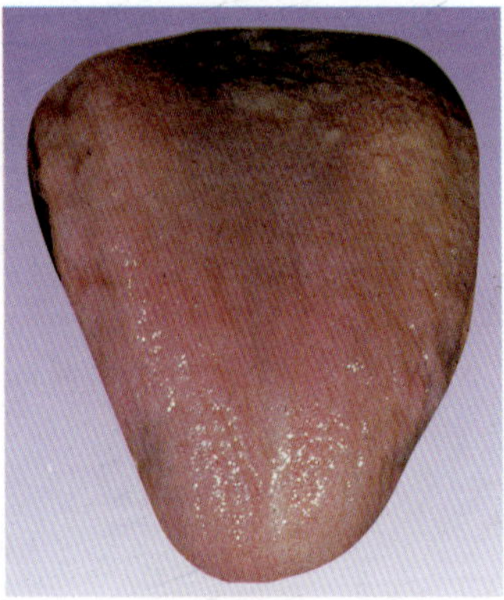

图7.9 淡白偏暗舌，根部浮垢苔

Figure 7.9 The Pale and Dim Tongue with Floating Fur at the Root

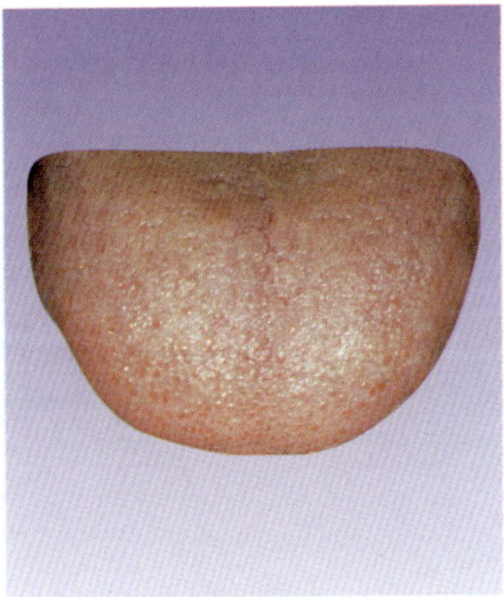

图 7.10 淡白红点舌，白腻中黄苔

Figure 7.10 The Pale Tongue with Red Spots, Covered by White and Sticky Fur, Showing Yellow Fur in The Middle Part

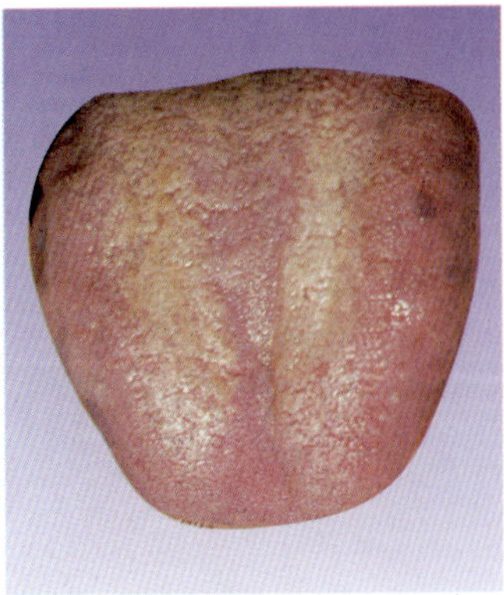

图 7.11 淡白瘀斑舌，双黄苔

Figure 7.11 The Pale and Petechia Tongue Covered by White Fur with Double Yellow Fur

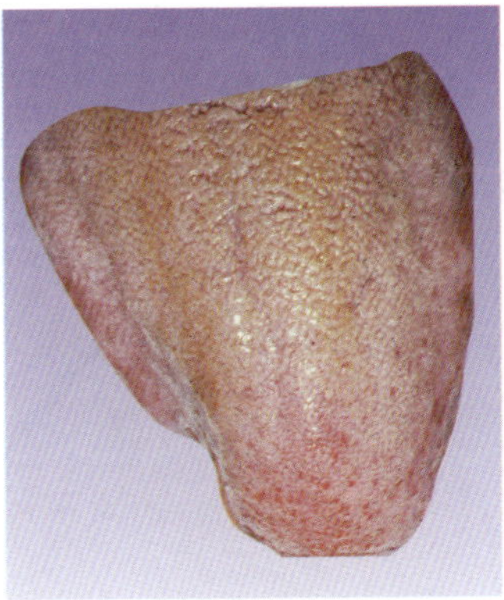

图 7.12 淡白齿痕舌，薄白双黄苔

Figure 7.12 The Pale Tongue with Tooth Traces, Covered by Thin and White Fur, Showing Double Yellow Coating on the Bilateral Sides

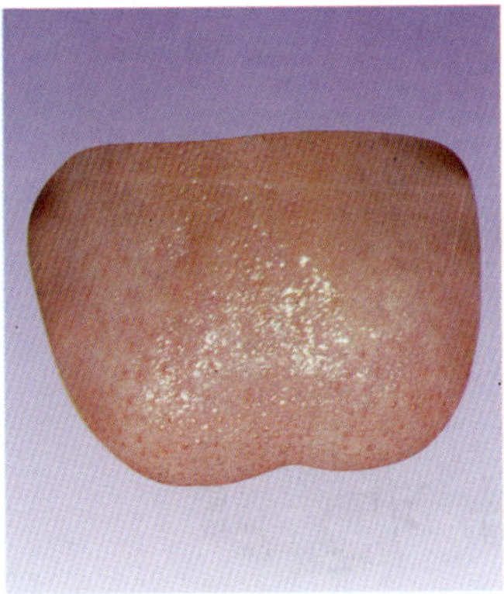

图 7.13 淡白偏暗舌，白腻双黄苔

Figure 7.13 The Pale and Dim Tongue Covered by White and Sticky Fur with Double Yellow Furs

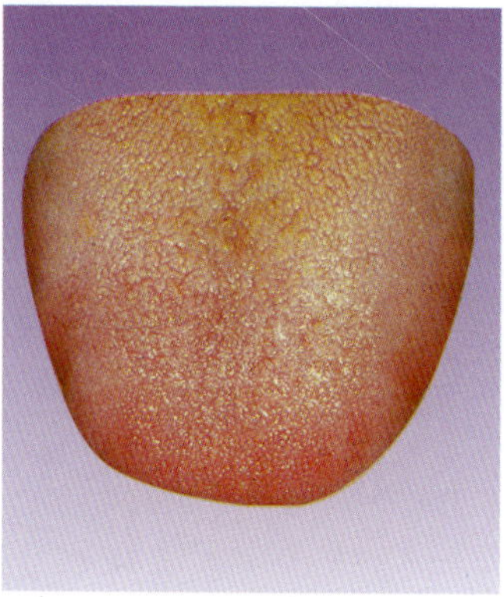

图7.14 淡白偏暗舌，白腻根黄苔

Figure 7.14 The White Pale and A Bit Dark Tongue Covered by Sticky and White, Yellow Fur at The Root

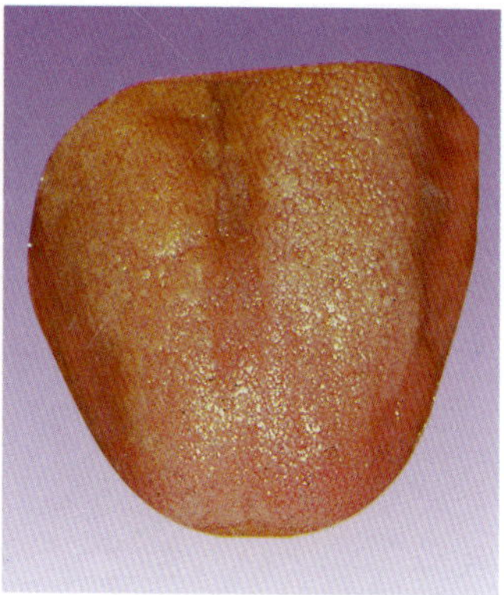

图7.15 淡白舌，白腻根黄苔

Figure 7.15 The Pale Tongue Covered by White and Sticky Fur with Yellow Appearance at the Root

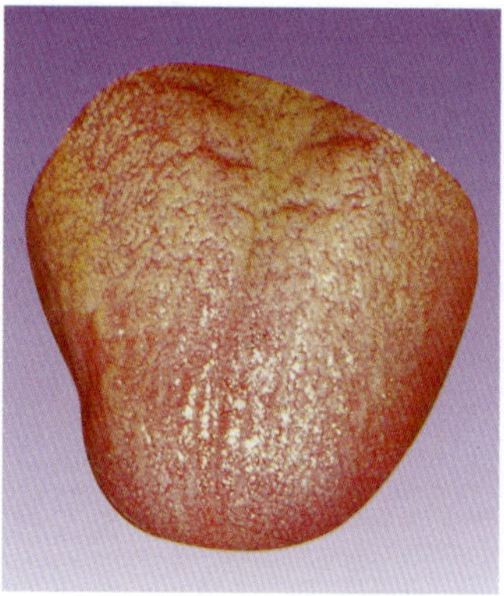

图7.16 淡白舌，白黄腻苔

Figure 7.16 The Pale Tongue with White, Yellow and Sticky Fur

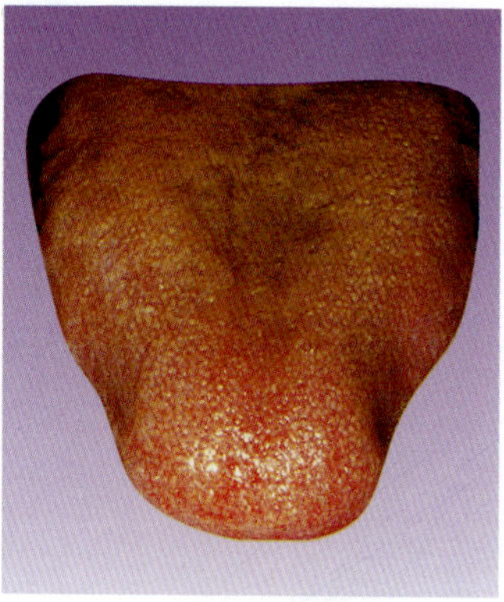

图7.17 淡白舌，黄腻苔

Figure 7.17 The Pale Tongue with Yellow and Sticky Fur

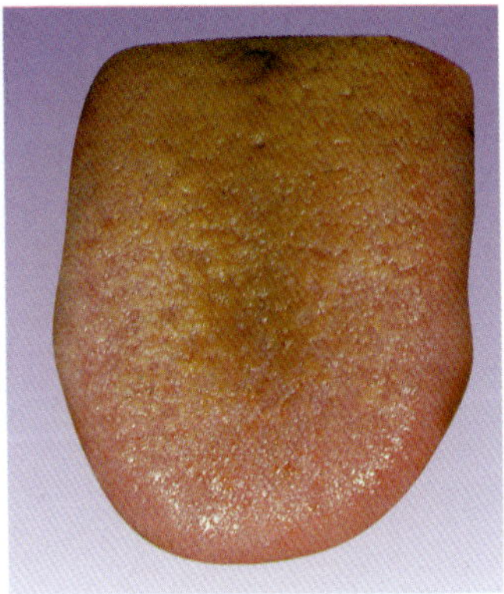

图7.18 淡白舌，白腻中灰苔
Figure 7.18 The Pale Tongue Covered by Sticky and White Fur with Gray Fur in the Middle

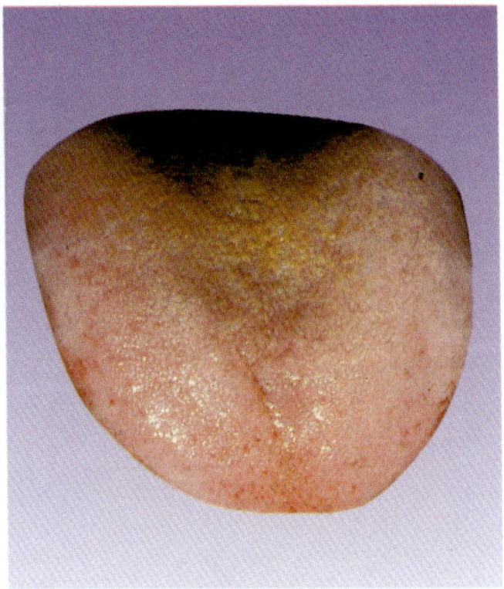

图7.19 淡白暗滞舌，根部黄灰苔
Figure 7.19 The Dim and Pale Tongue with Yellow and Gray Fur at the Root

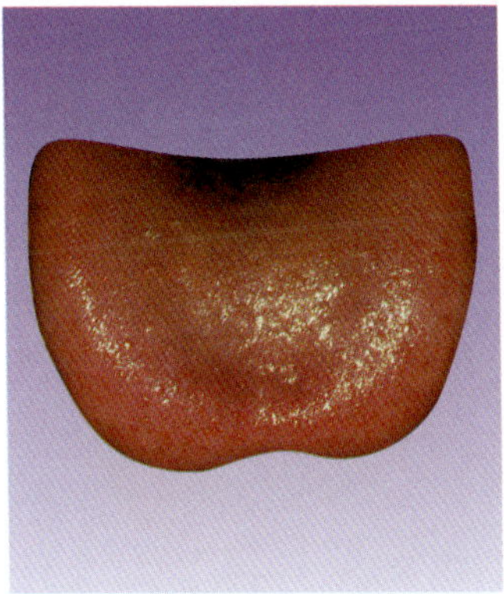

图8.1 淡红红点舌，薄白苔
Figure 8.1 The Reddish Tongue with Red Dots, Covered by Thin White Fur

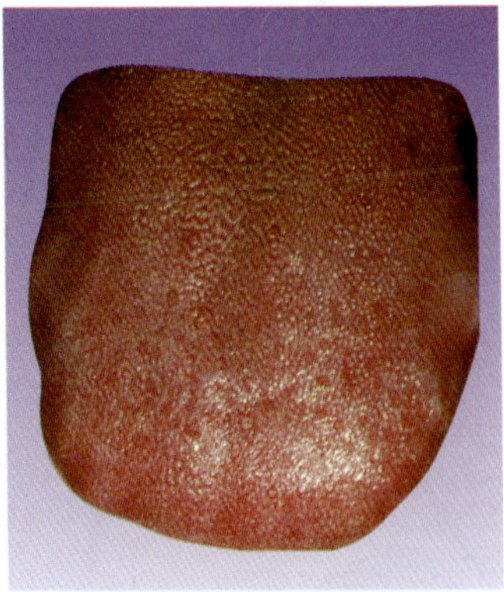

图8.2 淡红齿痕舌，薄白苔
Figure 8.2 The Reddish Tongue with Tooth-Prints Covered by Thin White Fur

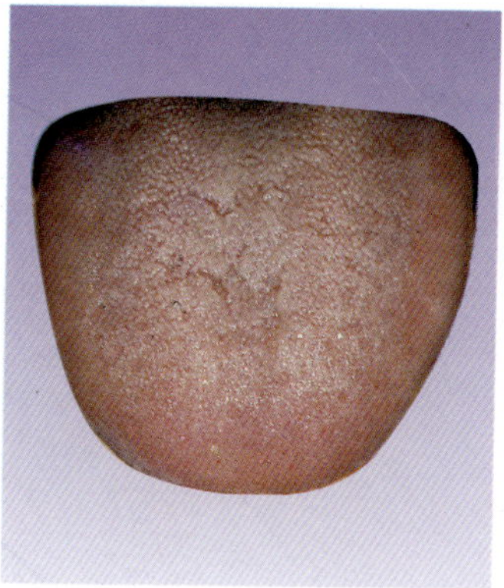

图8.3 淡红胖嫩舌，薄白干苔
Figure 8.3 The Reddish, Enlarhed and Tender Tongue, Covered by Thin, White and Dry Fur

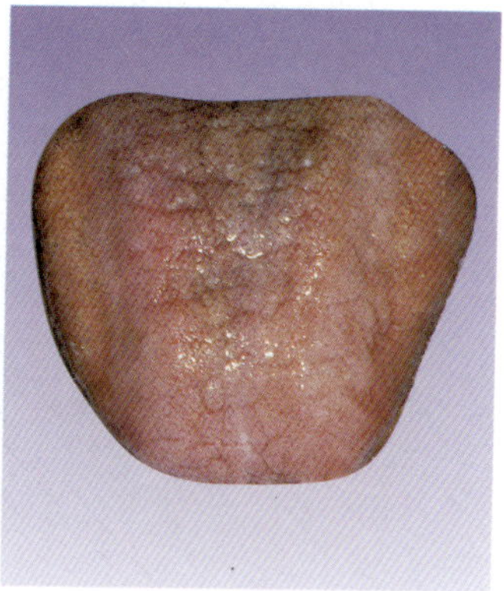

图8.4 淡红裂纹舌，透明苔
Figure 8.4 The Reddish Tongue with Fissures, Covered by Transparent Fur

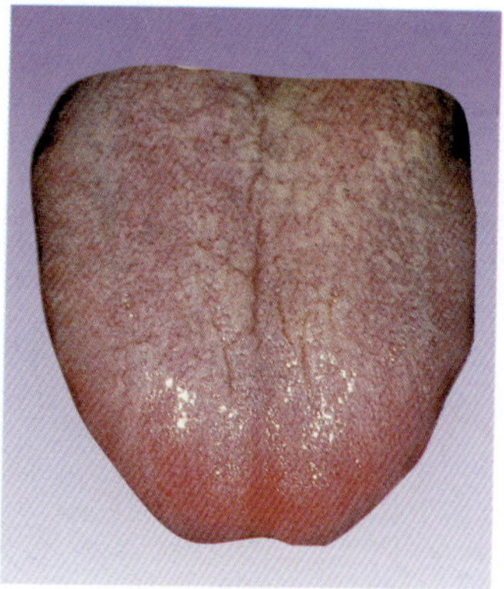

图8.5 淡红齿痕舌，白腻湿滑苔
Figure 8.5 The Reddish and Tooth Trace Tongue Covered by White, Sticky and Moist Fur

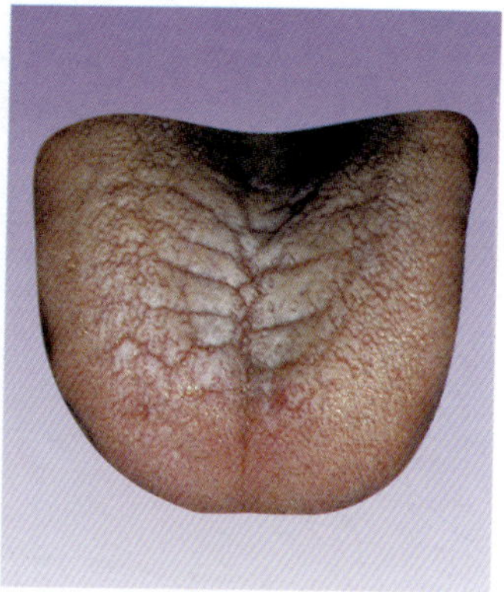

图8.6 淡红偏暗舌，白腐苔
Figure 8.6 The Reddish and Dim Tongue with Whiter and Curdy Fur

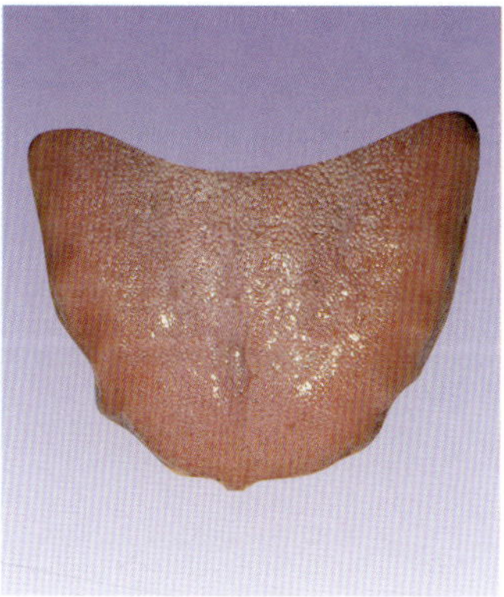

图8.7 淡红齿痕舌，薄白腻苔

Figure 8.7 The Reddish Tongue with Tooth Traces, Covered by Thin, White and Sticky Fur

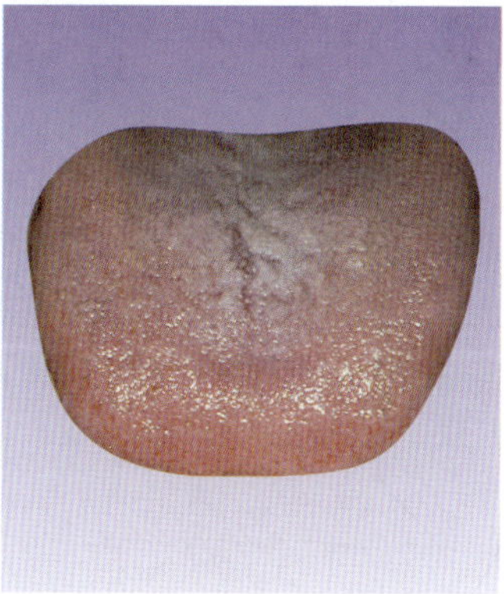

图8.8 淡红红点舌，白腐苔

Figure 8.8 The Reddish Tongue with Red Spots, Covered by White and Curdy Fur

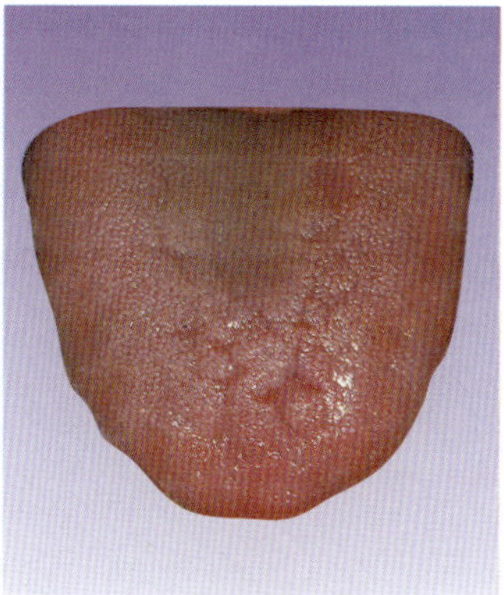

图8.9 淡红裂纹齿痕舌，中部淡黄苔

Figure 8.9 The Reddish Tongue Marked by Tooth Prints and Fissures, Covered with the Light Yellow and Sticky Fur in the Center

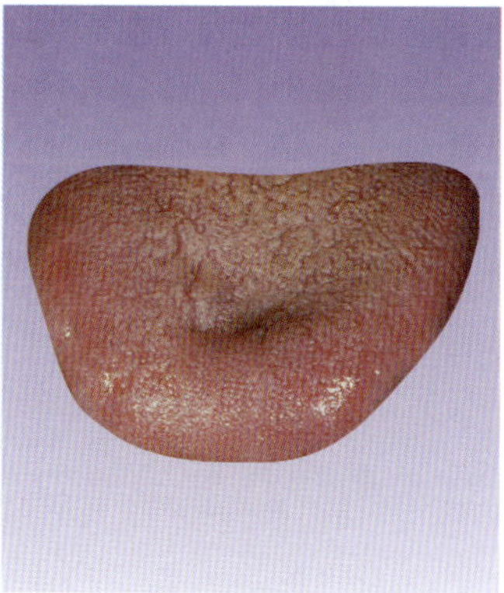

图8.10 淡红舌白腐淡黄苔

Figure 8.10 The Reddish Tongue Covered with Curdy White and Yellow Fur

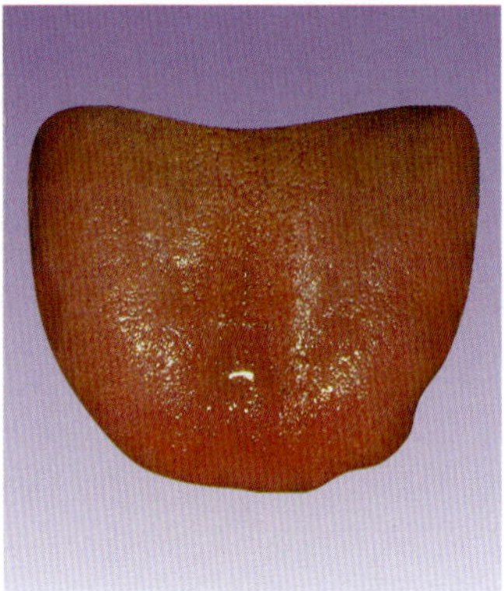

图 8.11 淡红红点舌，薄黄苔

Figure 8.11 The Reddish Tongue with Red Spots, Covered by Thin and Yellow Fur

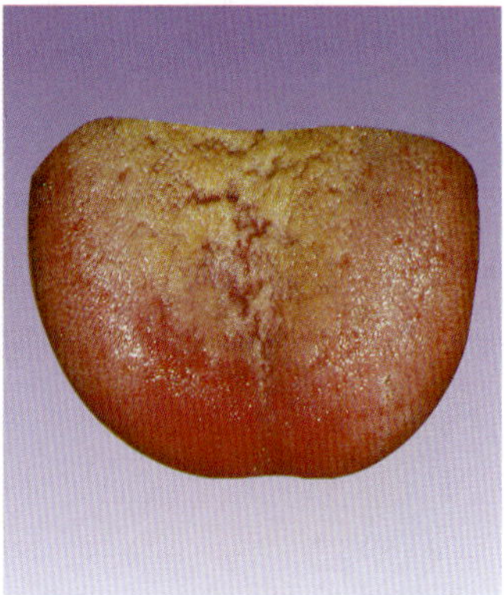

图 8.12 淡红偏暗舌，黄腻苔

Figure 8.12 The Reddish and Dim Tongue with Yellow and Sticky Fur

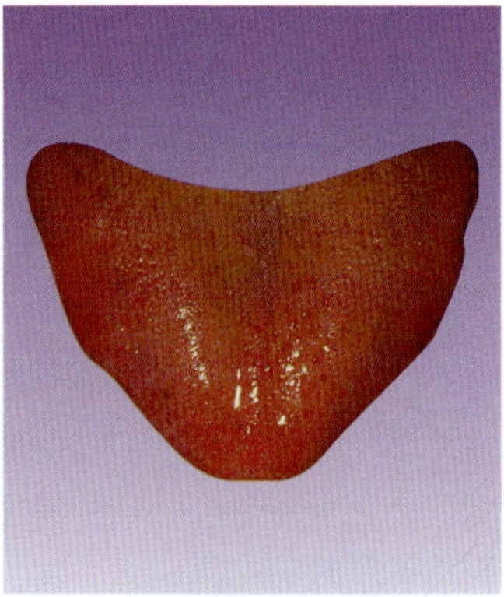

图 8.13 淡红瘀斑瘀点舌，薄黄腻苔

Figure 8.13 The Reddish Tongue with Petechia Covered by Thin, Yellow and Sticky Fur

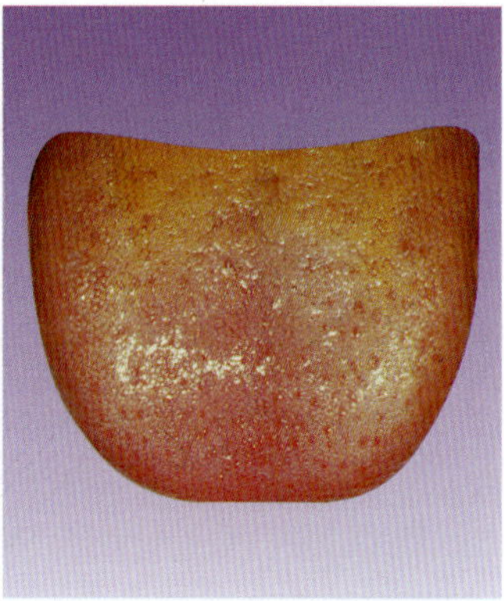

图 8.14 淡红舌，根黄腻苔

Figure 8.14 The Reddish Tongue with Yellow and Sticky Fur

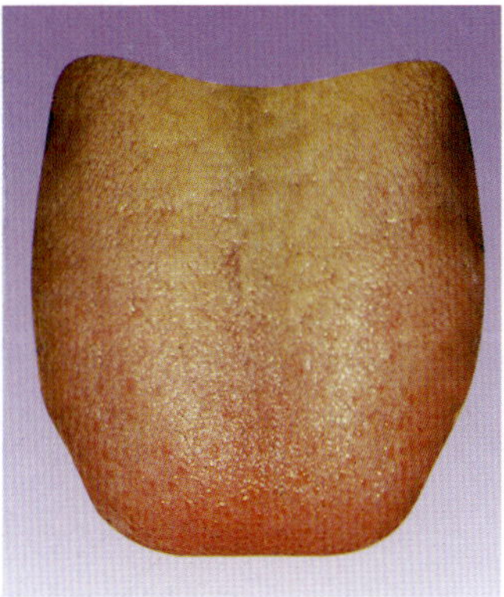

图 8.15 淡红红点舌，白腻淡黄苔

Figure 8.15 The Reddish Tongue with Red Dots, Covered by White, Sticky and Yellowish Fur

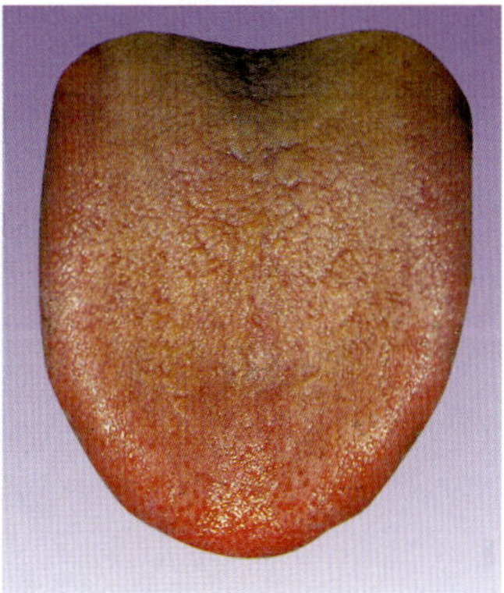

图 8.16 淡红尖红舌，淡黄干苔

Figure 8.16 The Reddish Tongue with Red Tip Covered by Yellowish and Dry Fur

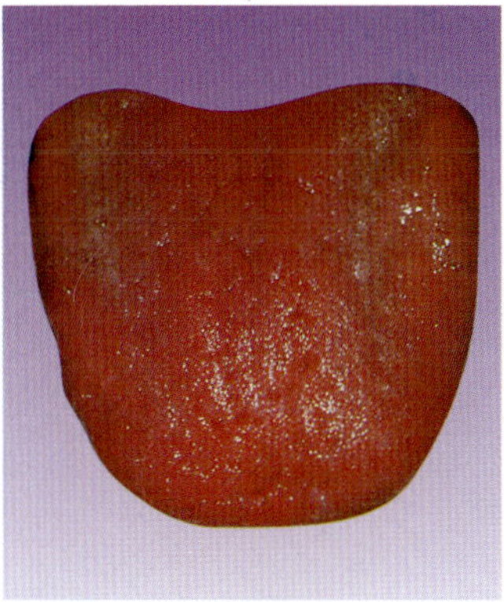

图 9.1 红光莹裂纹舌

Figure 9.1 The Red Glossy Tongue with Fissures

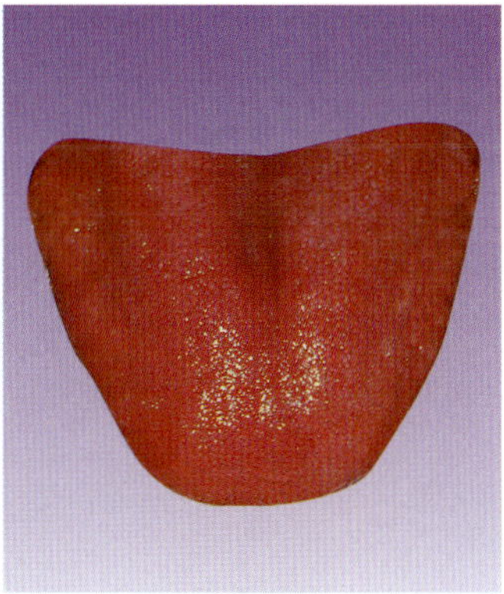

图 9.2 红嫩无苔舌

Figure 9.2 The Red and Tender Tongue without Fur

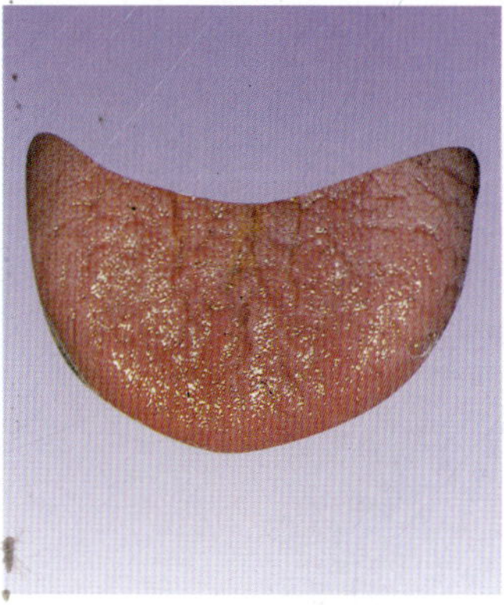

图 9.3 红瘦裂纹舌少苔
Figure 9.3 The Red and Thin Tongue with Fissures and Less Coating

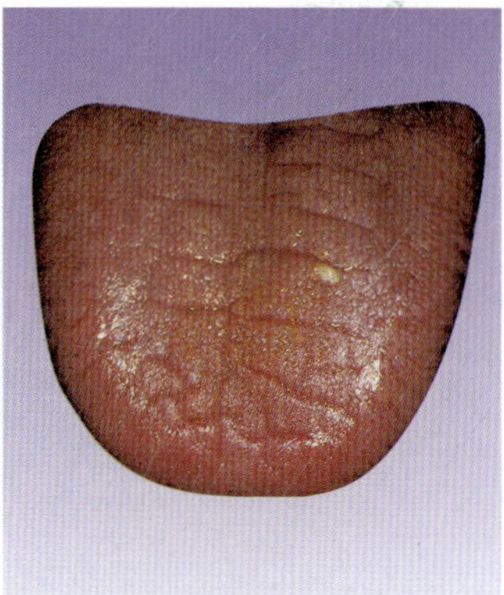

图 9.4 舌红少苔
Figure 9.4 The Red Tongue With Less Fur

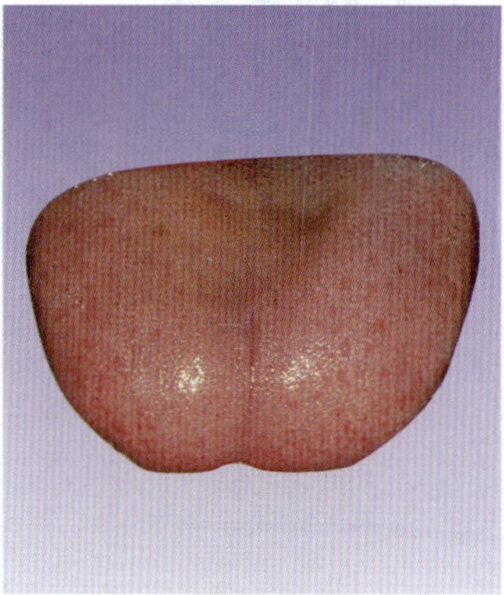

图 9.5 胖大红点舌少苔
Figure 9.5 The Enlarged Tongue with Red Dots and Less Fur

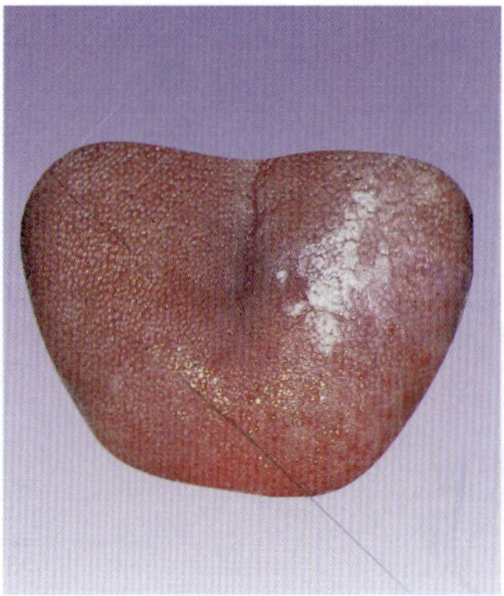

图 9.6 红舌类剥苔
Figure 9.6 The Red Tongue with Exfoliated Fur

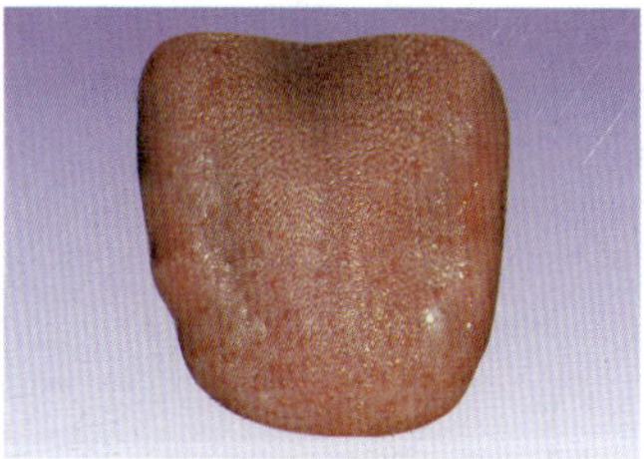

图 9.7 红夹红点舌少苔

Figure 9.7 The Red Tongue with Red Dots, Covered by Less Fur

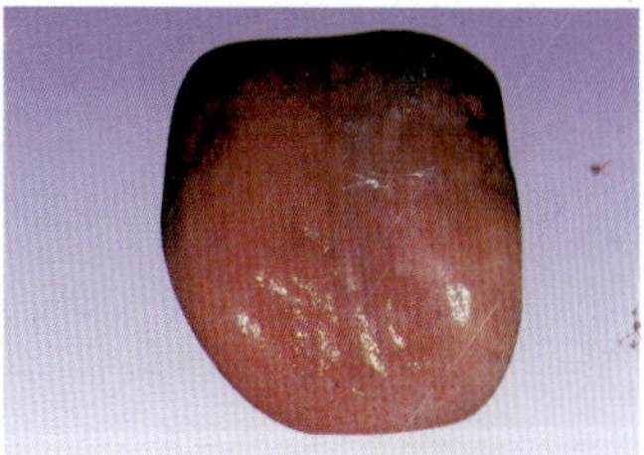

图 9.8 红嫩舌光剥苔

Figure 9.8 The Red and Tender Tongue without Fur

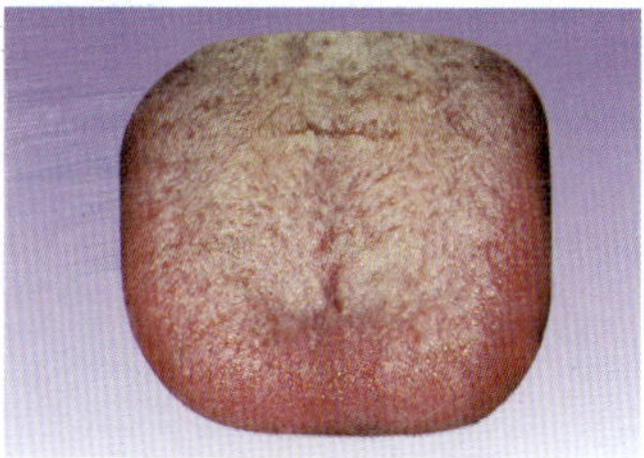

图 9.9 红偏暗舌白厚腻苔

Figure 9.9 The Dark Red Ton-gue with White and Sticky, Thick Fur

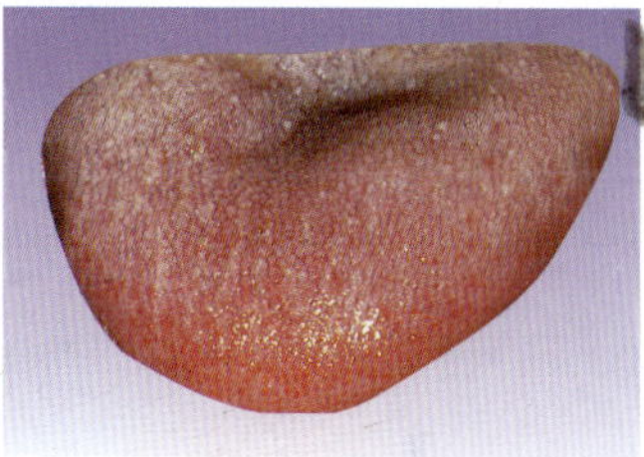

图 9.10 红点舌白腻苔

Figure 9.10 The Red Dotted Tongue with Sticky and White Fur

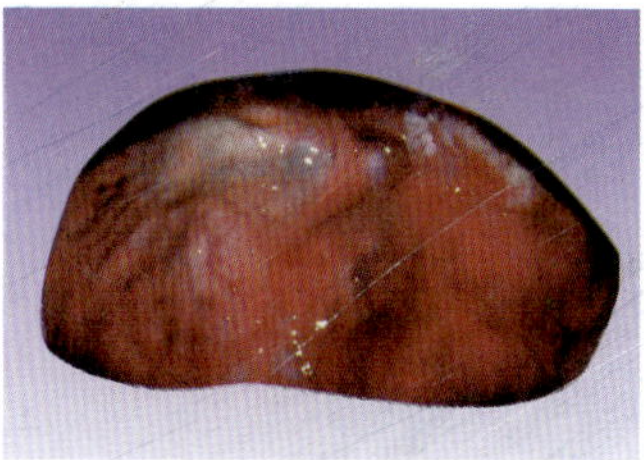

图 10.1 红绛裂纹无苔舌

Figure 10.1 The Crimson Tongue with Fissures and no Fur

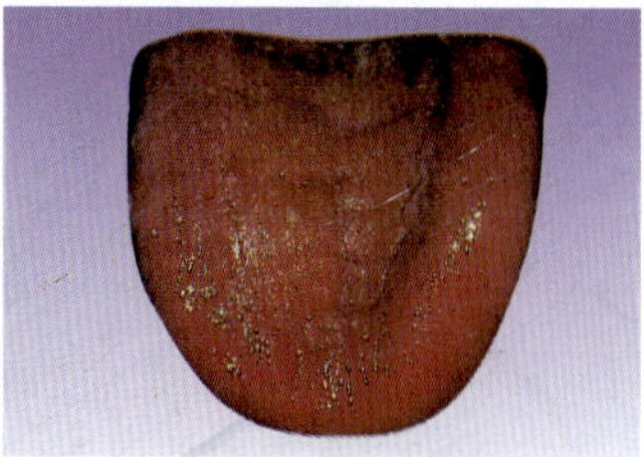

图 10.2 舌疮

Figure 10.2 The Ulcer of Tongue

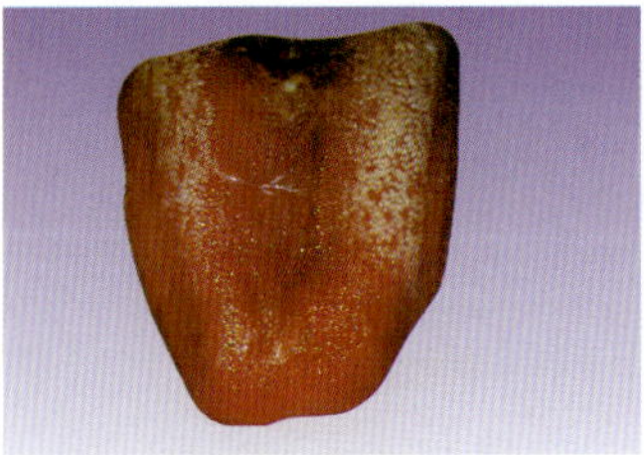

图 10.3 红绛舌中剥苔
Figure 10.3 The Crimson Tongue with Exfoliated Fur in the Middle

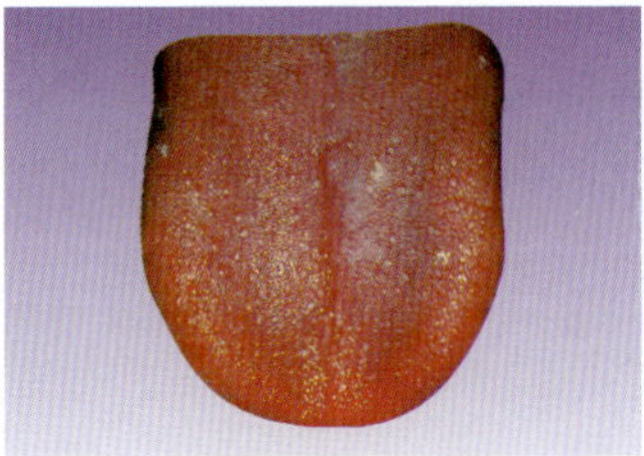

图 10.4 红绛芒刺舌，薄白少苔
Figure 10.4 The Red Tongue with Prickles and Less Thin and White Fur

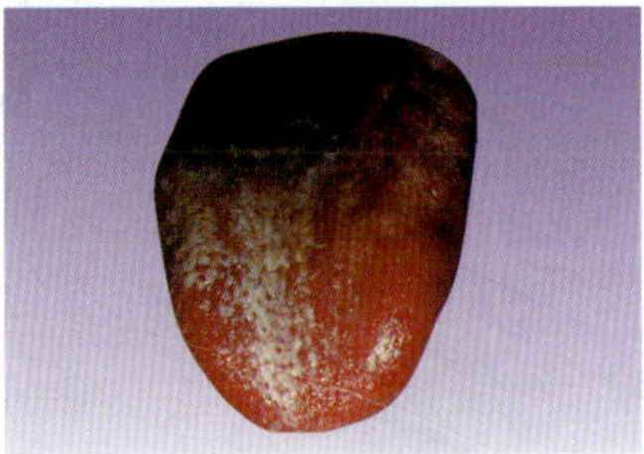

图 10.5 绛瘦舌，白腻花剥苔
Figure 10.5 The Crimson and Emaciated Tongue with White Sticky and Exfoliated Fur

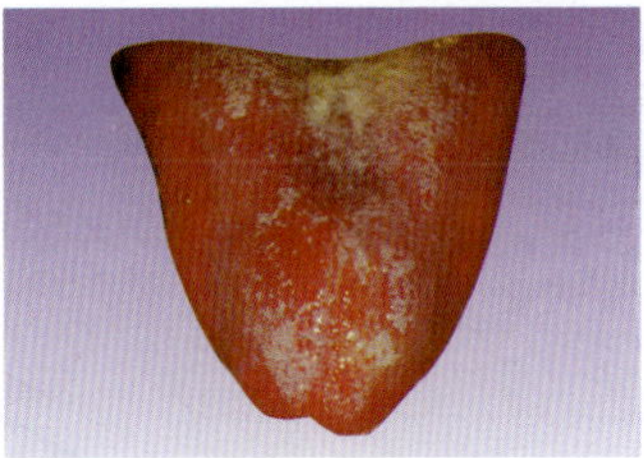

图 10.6 红瘦舌，白腻花剥苔
Figure 10.6 The Red and Thin Tongue with White, Sticky and Exfoliated Fur

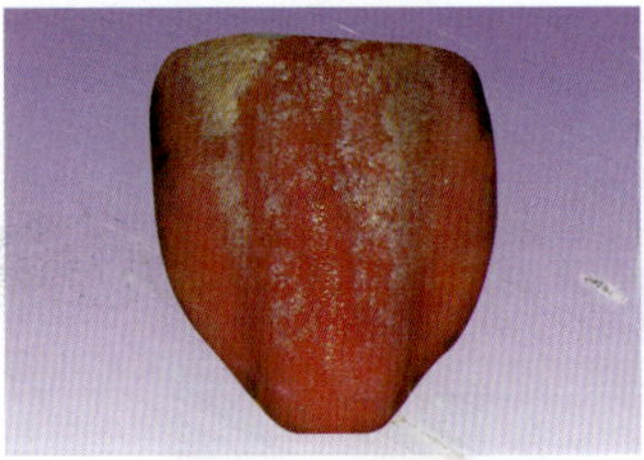

图 10.7 红绛舌，白腻花剥苔
Figure 10.7 The Crimson Tongue with White, Sticky and Exfoliated Fur

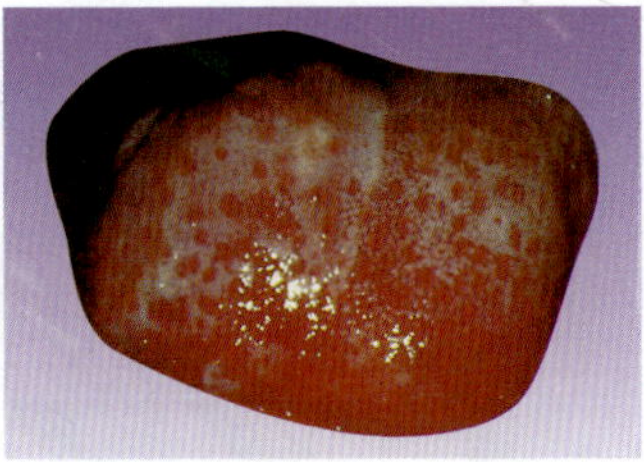

图 10.8 红绛红点舌，薄白腻滑苔
Figure 10.8 The Crimson Tongue with Red Dots, Covered by Thin, White, Sticky and Watery Fur

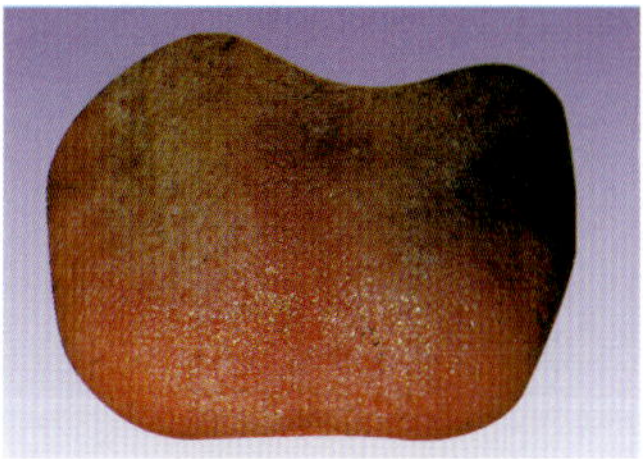

图 10.9 红绛舌，白腻淡黄苔
Figure 10.9 The Crimson Tongue with Sticky, White and Light Yellow Fur

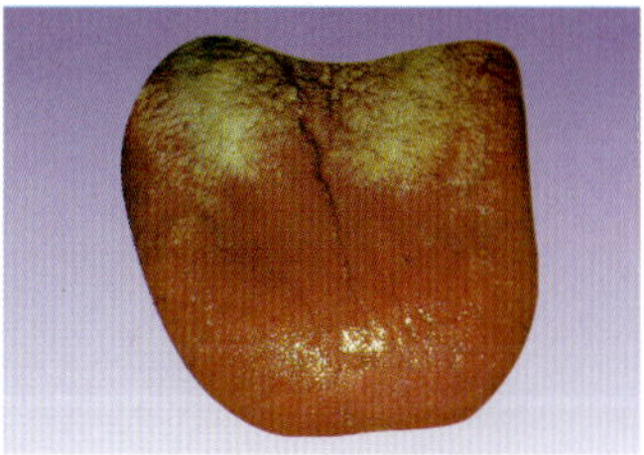

图 10.10 红绛肿胀舌，根黄腐苔
Figure 10.10 The Crimson and Swollen Tongue Covered by the Yellow and Curdy Fur at the Root

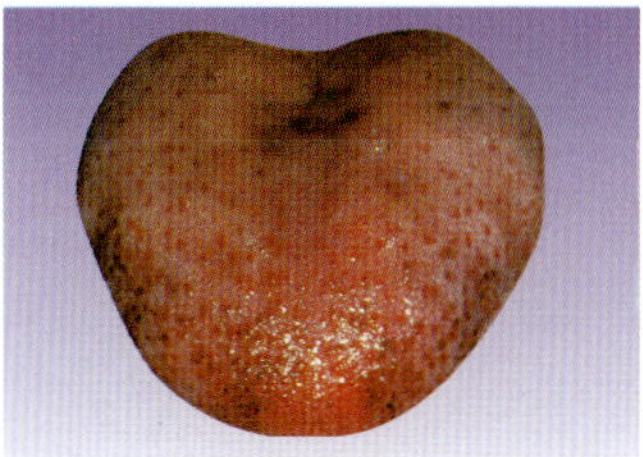

图 11.1 暗紫黑点舌，薄白透明苔
Figure 11.1 The Dark Purple Tongue with Black Dots Covered by the Thin, White and Clarity Coating

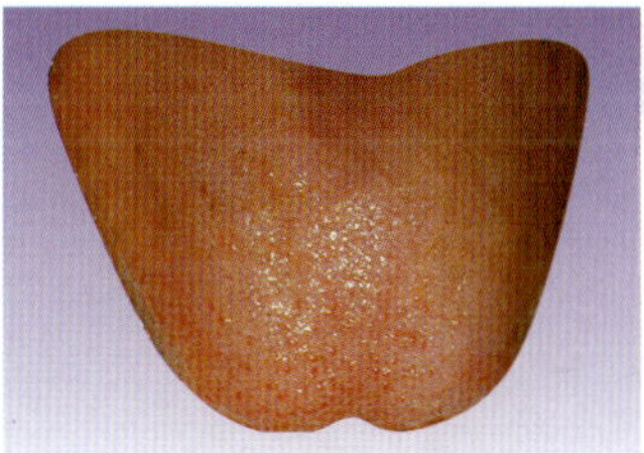

图 11.2 淡紫瘀点舌，透明苔
Figure 11.2 The Light Purple Tongue with Dark Spots Covered by Clarity Coating

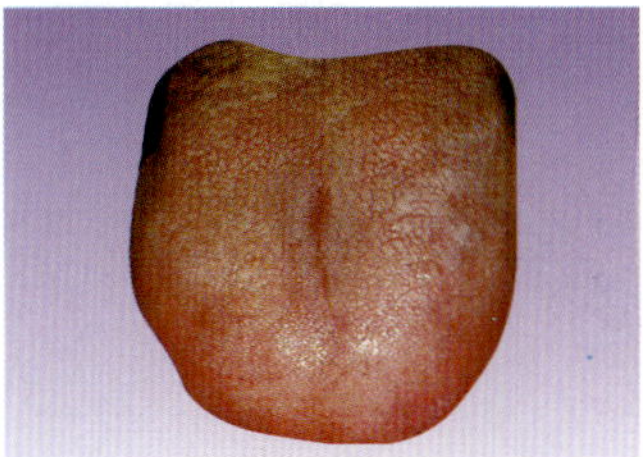

图 11.3 淡紫胖嫩舌，薄白润苔
Figure 11.3 The Purplish, Enlarged and Tender Tongue Covered by Thin Whiteness and Moist Coating

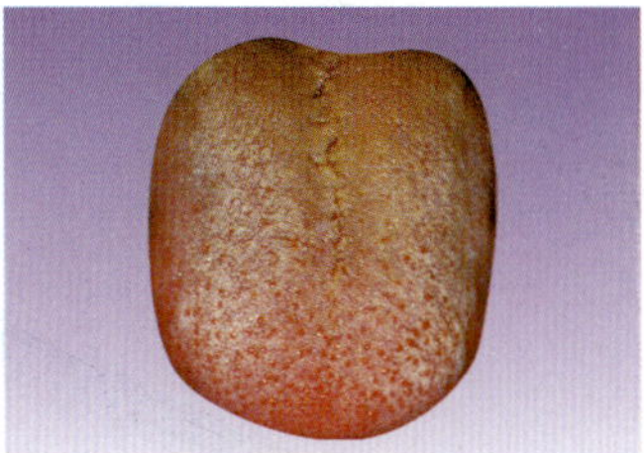

图 11.4 暗紫红点舌，白腻干苔
Figure 11.4 The Dark Purple Tongue with Some Red Dots Covered by White, Greasy and Dry Coating

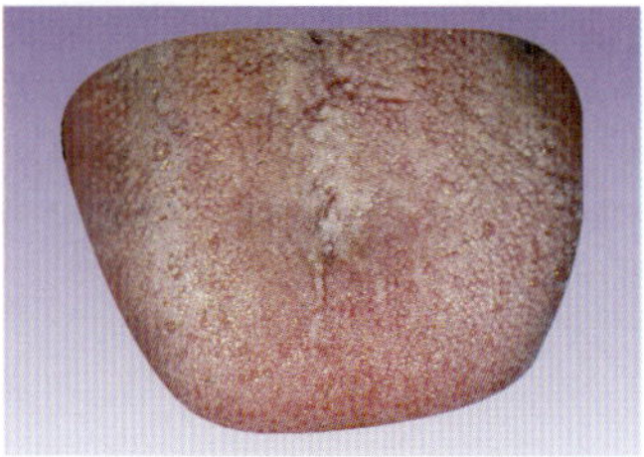

图 11.5 暗紫偏歪舌，白腻湿润苔
Figure 11.5 The Dark Purple and Deviated Tongue Covered by Wh-ite, Greasy and Moist Coating

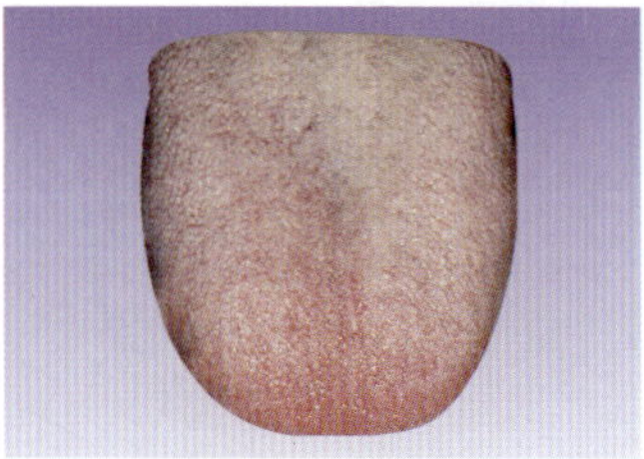

图 11.6 淡紫舌，薄白腻苔
Figure 11.6 The Purple To-ngue with White and Greasy Coating

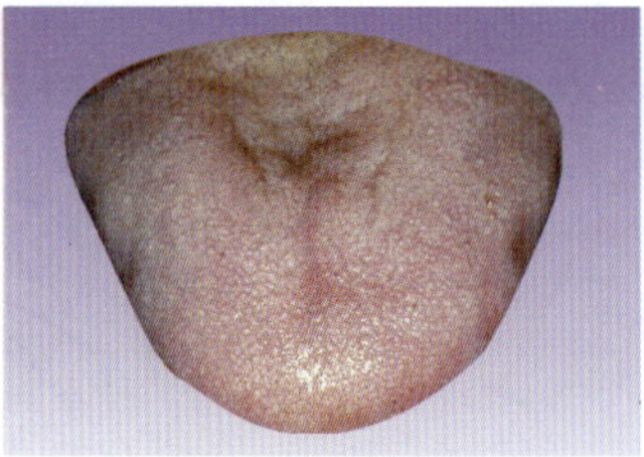

图 11.7 青紫淡嫩舌，薄白水滑苔
Figure 11.7 The Bluish Purple and Tender Tongue with Thin Whiteness and Watery Coating

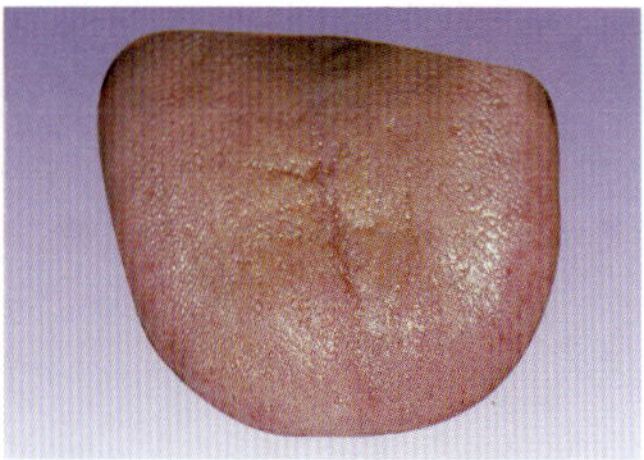

图 11.8 淡紫红点舌，白腻淡白苔
Figure 11.8 The Purplish To-ngue with Red Spots Covered by Greasy, White and Yel-lowish Coating

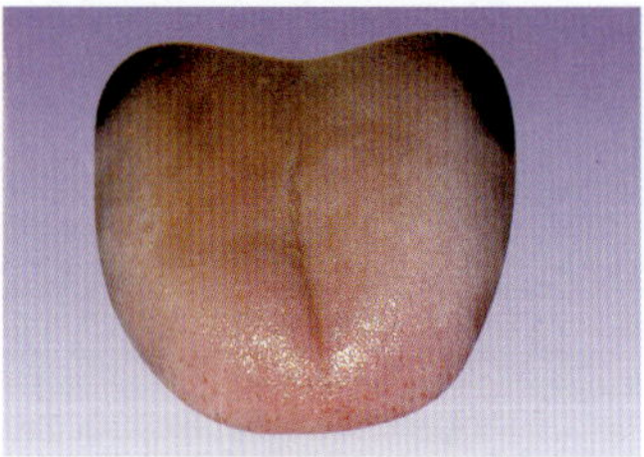

图 11.9 淡紫胖嫩舌，薄腻中灰苔
Figure 11.9 The Purple and Enlarged Tongue Covered by Thin and Greasy Coating Sh-owing Gray Fur in the Middle

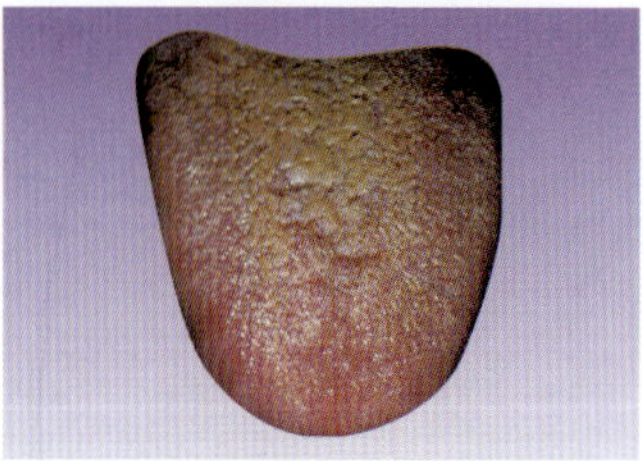

图 11.10 绛紫舌，黄腻燥裂苔
Figure 11.10 The Crimson Purple Tongue with Yellow, Greasy and Dryness Coating Showing Fissures